555

Ways to
Reward Your
Dental Team

Dr. Joe Blaes and Dr. Nate Booth

Printed in Canada

Harrison Acorn Press

Copyright © 2000 by Nate Booth

Designed and edited by Carlen Media Group, Sausalito, CA

First printing 2000
1 2   3   4   5   6   7   8   9   10
ISBN: 0-9649500-2-2

ATTENTION CORPORATIONS, UNIVERSITIES, COLLEGES AND PROFESSIONAL ORGANIZATIONS:
Quantity discounts are available on bulk purchases of this book for educational or training purposes. Special books or book excerpts can also be created to fit specific needs.

For more information, contact:
Harrison Acorn Press
227 N. El Camino Real, Suite 106
Encinitas, CA 92024
800.917.0008
www.natebooth.com
nbooth@natebooth.com

DEDICATION

This book is dedicated to the thousands of
hardworking people who support dentists and
their teams every day. Their dedication to
exceptional patient care is a vital component of
every practice's success. We hope this book
helps them feel more appreciated.

ACKNOWLEDGMENTS

The following people were instrumental in making this book a reality:

The dentists and their staffs who contributed many of the reward and recognition ideas presented in this book.

All the wonderful people at Fortune Practice Management, who provided ideas and support for the book.

Bob Nelson, the author of the book, *1001 Ways to Reward Employees*. Bob was very gracious with letting us use some of his key ideas. We strongly recommend his book to anyone working in a corporation.

Carlen Media Group, for providing stellar creative services, including cover design.

contents

Introduction

It's common sense to know that each member of your staff wants to feel appreciated. But common sense is not common practice in many dental offices today. How many dentists consider "appreciating my staff" to be a major function of their daily jobs? It should be. Dentists do care about the people they work with, but often they are too busy, too stressed or simply don't have enough good ideas to make their staff feel appreciated on a consistent basis.

There are two groups of people who walk into your office each day — your patients and your staff. Both groups are important. It's very easy to get totally preoccupied with serving your patients because there's a sense of urgency associated with them. ("We need to take great care of them now because they are only here for a short time, and they pay the bills.") Your staff is just as important, but there isn't that sense of urgency associated with them. ("They're here all the time, and they don't pay the bills.") Even though the urgency isn't there, you must consistently let your staff know how much you appreciate them with effective rewards.

555 Ways to Reward Your Dental Staff will be a valuable resource tool to help you do this! This book is loaded with 555 specific, effective and powerful ways you can acknowledge, praise, congratulate, thank, recognize and reward your office staff. When you do this on a consistent basis, you will create four results:

1. Rewards let your staff know that you care about them and are grateful for their efforts. Your people are aching to make a commitment to improve your practice. They only ask to be recognized for it. This

The deepest principle in human nature is the craving to be appreciated.
- William James

Gratitude is the heart's memory.
- French Proverb

is so important in today's world because high-tech needs to be balanced by an equal amount of high touch. Showing people your appreciation is the ultimate in high touch.

2. Rewards reinforce the kinds of behavior you want to see in your staff. As you remember from Psychology 101, any action that's followed by positive reinforcement is more likely to happen again. It has been said that the world's greatest management principle is, "You get what you reward."

    For clarity, I define a reward as any positive reinforcement. A recognition is a reward that does not involve the giving of something material – for example, a compliment. Your staff is aching to make a commitment to improve your practice. They only ask to be recognized for it.

3. Rewards help create a team that is happy, focused and productive. You can tell a lot about a dental office when you walk in the door. Some practices feel cold and impersonal. Others radiate warmth and caring. The way you treat your staff is going to set the tone for how they treat each other and your patients. You don't get satisfied patients without first having satisfied employees. It all begins with you, and implementing a well-constructed reward program is a great place for you to begin.

    An effective reward program is "the right thing to do," and it will have a direct, bottom-line impact in your practice. Implementing such a practice has been proven to decrease costs and increase revenue. Rewards decrease stress, absenteeism and turnover. It increases morale and productivity. Consequently, profits rise.

It's not what we have, but what we give, that brings joy.
- Author unknown

4. Rewarding others will enhance your life. As you will learn in Chapter 8, giving will energize your Cycle of Life, allowing you to be, do, have and give even more.

Here's a brief overview of what you will learn in this book. In Chapter 1, you will learn why a well-planned recognition and reward system is vital to your practice's success. In Chapter 2, you will learn how to elegantly compliment and recognize your staff on a regular basis. In Chapters 3 through 6, you will learn hundreds of cost-effective ways you can reward your staff with merchandise, food, clothing, money, gift certificates, awards and time off. In Chapter 7, I will show you how to construct a creative incentive plan that inspires the actions and results you want. In Chapter 8, you will learn why giving will ignite a powerful cycle of success for everyone involved. In Chapter 9, you will create a formal reward program that fits your budget and practice philosophy. In Chapter 10, you will learn how to refine your reward program. You will also find Appendix A extremely valuable. It contains a list of companies from which you can obtain a wide variety of reward items.

This book is loaded with practical reward ideas you can use today to make your office a more enjoyable and profitable place. Many of the ideas have come from dozens of dental practices like yours. Practices like Dr. Marty Kolinski's in St. Charles, Illinois. Here's what Dr. Kolinski says about the value of an effective recognition and reward program.

"We take great pride in our office's TEAM APPROACH. Our staff is highly self-motivated and independent. We attribute some of these qualities to the feeling of value that the staff has. The most important thing we have done for the staff is to be sure they are well educated — not only in what they do, but in what every person on the dental team does, and why they do it. This allows each staff member to feel confident and of value to the team."

Here's how I recommend you use this book. Read it through completely, cover-to-cover. I have purposefully created this book to be a buffet of reward ideas. Just select the ideas that appeal to you now. Leave the rest of them on the buffet table for a future "meal."

Make your buffet selections by putting a big check mark in front of all the recognition and reward ideas that work for you. Also, in the margins and in the spaces designated, write all the ideas the material sparks in your mind. In Chapter 9, you will use all of this information to create a customized reward plan that complements your personal and practice philosophies and creates the outcomes you want to achieve.

DO NOT put this book on some out-of-the-way bookshelf. Keep *555 Ways to Reward Your Dental Staff* in the top drawer of your office desk. Refer to it regularly for fresh reward ideas to help build the practice you desire and deserve!

It's time to get started on your reward program that will let your staff know how much you appreciate them. Turn to Chapter 1 right now and learn about . . . **Recognition and Reward: An Essential Component of Your Success**.

1 | Recognition & Reward: An Essential Component of Success

Principles of which you are unaware hold you prisoner. There are dozens of these principles exerting their power over your dental practice right now. They're like huge waves in the ocean. Are you going to:

1. Ignore the waves and have your boat capsized?

2. Fight the waves and have your boat destroyed?

3. Identify the waves, start rowing and ride the waves to the practice of your dreams?

This book is based on one of these powerful waves – a wave that, when you truly understand and harness, will carry your entire office to emotional and financial success. The principle is that people act in ways that give them pleasure. The rewards in this book are the pleasure you can provide to your staff. Simple, isn't it? But don't let the simplicity fool you. There is tremendous and easily accessible power in this information when you consistently and effectively apply it in your dental practice.

The trouble with man is twofold: He cannot learn truths which are too complicated; and he forgets truths which are too simple.
- Rebecca West

So what pleasure do people want from their jobs? A series of studies done by Lawrence Lindahl, Ken Kovach and Bob Nelson discovered that what managers perceived as being most important to employees differed vastly from what the employees reported as being desirable. Following is a chart of ten factors people could desire in a job, and how managers and employees ranked each from 1 to 10, 1 being the most desirable.

Factor	Managers	Employees
Good wages	1	5
Job security	2	4
Promotion/growth opportunities	3	7
Good working conditions	4	9
Interesting work	5	6
Personal loyalty to employees	6	8
Tactful disciplining	7	10
Full appreciation of work done	8	1
Sympathetic to personal problems	9	3
Feeling "in" on things	10	2

As you can see from the scores above, managers thought money would be ranked the highest. Employees ranked "full appreciation of work done" as most desirable. Their managers ranked it eighth!

In another recent national survey by the staffing firm Robert Half International, "limited recognition and praise" was cited as the most common reason why employees left a company. It was ranked higher than compensation and personality conflicts.

Some doctors might ask, "Why isn't what I pay my staff good enough to get them to do their job? Why do I have to do more?" People will do their jobs for what they get paid, but they won't do their best job – and isn't that what you want? The extra effort that it takes to move from "doing my job" to "doing my best job" is directly related to how people are treated, not what they are paid.

In addition to helping people do their best work, rewards are vital to your professional practice for five other reasons:

1. As baby boomers get older and retire from the workforce, fewer qualified people will be available to work in your practice. The practices that are "staff-friendly" will retain and attract high-quality people more effectively.

2. Younger staff members have different values than their parents. They expect their workplace to be motivating and personally rewarding.

3. Coercion doesn't work with today's professional staffs. Increasingly, you must be a coach who influences behavior with positive reinforcement.

4. With the increased levels of responsibility in dental practices today, you must create an office environment that is supportive and reinforcing so that people take initiative on their own.

5. In an era when your bottom line is getting squeezed from various directions, an effective rewards program will increase your ROP (Return On People). The salaries you pay your staff may be the biggest expense you have. Investing in rewarding them is "the right thing to do" and it makes good business sense.

So how often are today's employees receiving the rewards they desire? Take a look at these statistics taken from a study done by Dr. Gerald Graham of 1500 corporate employees:

- **58 percent** said they seldom if ever received personal thanks from their manager

- **76 percent** said they seldom if ever received written thanks from their manager

- **81 percent** said they seldom if ever received public praise in the workplace

- **92 percent** said they seldom if ever participated in morale-building meetings

After looking at the statistics presented in this chapter, there is one important conclusion you can make – the reward techniques that have the greatest impact are practiced the least even though they are easier and less expensive to use. Simple gestures count the most!

Rewards come in all shapes and sizes. They can be formal (part of a planned program) or informal (given spontaneously). They can be free (a warm smile and a sincere "thank you"), simple (a single red rose in a bud vase for each staff member at the end of a productive day) or elaborate (a team trip to Bermuda). Rewards also can be part of a creative compensation plan that recognizes people for results. The rewards can be given on a fixed schedule (a quarterly bonus) or a variable schedule (a surprise afternoon off). Remember, the most effective positive reinforcement is often the most simple and least expensive.

The happiness of life is made up of minute fractions. . . The little soon forgotten charities of a kiss or smile, a kind look, a heartfelt compliment, and the countless infinitesimals of pleasurable and genial feeling.
- Samuel Taylor Coleridge

Nine Guidelines for Rewarding Your Staff

1. *Match the reward to the staff member.* What may be a reward for one person may not be a reward for another person. The following are three ways you can discover the unique rewards for a person:

   a. Watch people's reaction when you reward them. They will verbally and nonverbally communicate the rewards that excite them the most.
   b. Listen to people's conversations. They will give you clues as to what they uniquely desire.
   c. Ask other team members what would be great rewards for their teammates.

   In addition, ask yourself the following questions:

   - Do they have any hobbies, such as woodworking, furniture refinishing, crafts, gardening or cooking?
   - Do they have any special interests, such as card games, theater, music or museums?
   - Do they speak another language?
   - Do they play a musical instrument or sing?
   - Do they like to draw, paint or cartoon?
   - What books, movies and music do they like?
   - What are their favorite sports?
   - What organizations and clubs do they belong to?
   - What causes are they interested in?

   Now create a file with the information you've collected for each staff member. Add to the file as you discover additional information.

2. *Match the reward to the action or achievement.* Use smaller rewards for smaller actions or achievements. Use larger rewards for larger achievements. It's important to remember that the amount of money a reward costs isn't the only thing that determines its size. A sincere pat-on-the-back can be more powerful than a $1,000 bonus. You will learn more about this vital concept in Chapter 2.

3. *Be specific.* Always communicate why the reward is given so people can solidly connect their behavior to the reward's pleasure. This is a concept that often gets overlooked. It's vital that the reward be tied to a specific event, situation or time. As an example, "Sally, I just

Men and women want to do a good job, a creative job, and if they are provided the proper environment, they will do so.
- Bill Hewlett, co-founder, Hewlett-Packard, from *1001 Ways to Reward Employees*

wanted you to know how much I appreciate how well you took care of Mrs. Jones today. She was very nervous at the beginning of her appointment. When you told her that joke, it really relaxed her and me. The procedure went very smoothly thanks to you. Keep up the great work!"

Do you see how this is more impactful than just saying, "Sally, I want to thank you for the good work you did last Tuesday"? It's crucial that the person being acknowledged really "gets it" – that they solidly connect the praise with the specific deed.

4. *Be timely.* Give the reward as soon as possible after the action or achievement is done. Long time lags decrease the power of the reward.

5. *Use fixed AND variable rewards.* If you use the same fixed rewards over and over again, it becomes boring at best and expected at worst. Here's a great example of this in action. How long would you stay at a casino slot machine if you won a penny every time you pulled the handle? It might be a little fun at first, but after a while it would be like having a job, right? Unless you were really poor, you would stop pulling the handle, which means the penny reward would lose its power.

The same is true of fixed rewards in your dental office – a $200 bonus every quarter, a turkey every Thanksgiving, or Christmas Eve Day off every December. I'm not saying stop doing these. Just realize that, after a while, these rewards lose most of their effectiveness. They can even create resentment if you stop giving them. I saw this happen in a company where I used to work. Every Christmas we received a $1,000 bonus. One year, when times were a little tough, we only received a $200 bonus. People were disappointed! The only thing most of them felt was the $800 they didn't receive.

Let's go back to our slot machine example. Why are slot machines so popular? It's because they pay off intermittently at unexpected times. You will want to do the same in your office. Every once in a while recognize a specific person or the entire office out of the blue. Every once in a while, spontaneously reward a specific person or the entire group with something that is totally unexpected.

It is one of the most beautiful compensations of this life that no man can sincerely try to help another without helping himself.
- Ralph Waldo Emerson, from
1001 Ways to Reward Employees

6. *Change your reward program frequently.* Variety is the spice of life. You will want to vary the who, what, when, where and why of your program.

    Who: Vary to whom you give the rewards. Sometimes reward the entire team, sometimes reward a team member for an act, an achievement or a result he or she created. Two weeks later reward another team member.

    Why: Vary the reasons why you give rewards. Sometimes recognize your team for no specific reason at all or just because you appreciate them. Sometimes recognize a team member for a single act of kindness towards a patient. Sometimes reward the entire team for one day of effort that was "above and beyond the call of duty." Sometimes reward the team members with a small gift for a good month of production. Sometimes reward the team for lowering expenses for a quarter by 6 percent. Sometimes reward the entire team with a two-day trip to a resort destination for achieving your production goals for the year. The number of "whys" you can recognize and reward is limited only by your imagination.

    What: Vary the kinds of rewards used. This book is filled with fresh ideas for recognizing your staff. Use the ideas presented here or create your own.

    When: Vary the times you reward. Don't become predictable.

    Where: Vary the location where the reward is given – sometimes have flowers sent to the office for a team member. Sometimes have flowers sent to a team member's home. Sometimes have flowers sent to a restaurant for a team member.

7. *Wrap every reward with emotion.* This will multiply the effect of the reward a hundred times. In word and deed let your staff know how much you appreciate them and value their contribution to the practice's success. It'll make you feel better too!

8. *Create a formal reward program.* If you're like most professionals, you see the value of a reward program, but you may lack the time and/or creativity to effectively execute one on a regular basis. That's why this book will be so valuable to you. It will be a quick and easy resource to help you create a reward program that matches your

It's up to you to decide how to speak to your people. Do you single out individuals for public praise and recognition? Make people who work for you feel important. If you honor and serve them, they'll honor and serve you.
- Mary Kay Ash, founder, Mary Kay Cosmetics, from *1001 Ways to Reward Employees*

values and your staff's desires – a program that will produce the emotional and financial results you want for your staff and yourself. Don't leave your reward program to chance, or it may not get done. In Chapter 10, you will construct a program that will create your office culture and produce the results you desire.

9. ***Begin with the end in mind.*** It's not always advisable to start at the beginning. Many times it's best to begin at the end. Before you commence your rewards program, crystallize in your mind the kind of practice you want to create. This is your dream practice. Now, your dream practice will be a beacon of light that will guide you in developing your reward program. Remember, whatever you praise, you increase. Identify the steps that will move you closer to your dream and reward the people who take those steps. When you do this, you will look at your reward program as a business strategy, not as a way to pay people.

Dr. Martin Luther King proclaimed, "I have a dream!" He didn't say, "I have a strategic plan." He didn't say, "I have an office manual." Dr. King began with the end. Then he laid out his plan for racial equality.

Walt Disney didn't want to have a company that made cartoons for kids. He wanted to create a company that would, "Use imagination to bring happiness to millions!" How would you like to work for a company like that? Walt's dream (the end he wanted to create in the future) directed his company's actions in the present.

Mary Kay Ash didn't want to start a company that would sell cosmetics to women. She wanted to create an organization that would provide tremendous opportunities for women. A company that would allow women to go as far as their talents and abilities would take them. She started with the end in mind. Then she took the appropriate actions that enabled her to enroll tens of thousands of other women who had similar dreams.

What is your dream for your dental practice? If you haven't thought about it in a while, maybe now would be a good time. What will the culture be like? How many people will be on your team? How will the team members be treating each other? How will the team members be treating the patients? How many active patients will you have? What kinds of care will you be providing? What quality of care will

The hard stuff is easy.
The soft stuff is hard.
And the soft stuff is a lot more important than the hard stuff.
- Milliken & Company slogan

you be providing? How much care will you be providing? How will everyone feel at the end of the day? What will be the financial rewards for you and your staff?

Take a minute or two right now to envision your dream practice. Shut this book and let your mind soar. Let the above questions stimulate your thinking. Don't be realistic. Realistic people accurately see the way things are now. Unrealistic people have compelling visions of the future. They dream things and ask, "Why not?" All progress is made by unrealistic people.

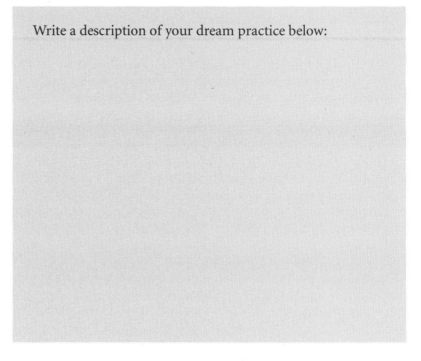

Write a description of your dream practice below:

Now that you have your dream practice embedded in your mind, as well as in the space above, you need to do two things:

a. *Communicate the dream to your staff.* Vividly and passionately let them know what you're committed to creating. Ask for their help and ideas in creating it, and construct a plan for them to share the rewards of the creation (see Chapter 7).

b. *Answer this question:* What actions and outcomes will move you toward that dream practice? These are the actions and outcomes you will want to reward. What are some intermediate goals your dental team needs to achieve on the way to your dream practice? These are the goals you will want to reward when reached. Write these actions and outcomes in the space below:

The bottom line is this: Crystallize your dream practice in your mind. Mental creation precedes physical creation. Then communicate your dream to your staff. Finally, provide copious amounts of rewards to your team every step of the way.

Don't wait for the dream to be totally achieved.

Reward steps along the way.

Let me close this chapter with one final thought. In addition to your reward program, you need to be a model of the behavior you want to see from your people. If you want your staff to treat your patients with kindness and respect, you must first treat your staff with kindness and respect. You must become the change you seek in your dental practice!

Take a second now to review this chapter. What ideas has it stimulated? What actions are you committed to taking in your practice? Write your answers in the space below.

Enough of the background information, let's get started with the 555 specific ways you can reward your dental staff. Move on to Chapter 2, and learn the power of **Compliments and Recognition**.

2 | Compliments & Recognition

The following chapter is one of the most important chapters in the emtire book because the most effective forms of reward cost next to nothing. A sincere thank you or a word of praise to your staff can mean more to them than a pay raise or a gift. The power comes from the fact that staff members know you noticed what they did, took the time to talk with them and then personally and quickly delivered the praise.

Numerous studies have demonstrated the power of praise. In one study done by Dr. Gerald Graham, the most powerful employee motivator was personalized, instant recognition from their manager! Following are the top five motivating techniques from Dr. Graham's study:

1. The manager personally congratulates employees who do a good job.

2. The manager writes personal notes about good performance.

3. The organization uses performance as the basis for promotion.

4. The manager publicly recognizes employees for good performance.

5. The manager holds morale-building meetings to celebrate successes.

As you can see, three of the five listed items above cost nothing, one involves a small monetary investment and one involves a larger monetary investment. When it comes to recognition and reward, it's the little things that make a big difference in motivating your staff. Praising people is the right thing to do and it's a sound business decision because you're investing in one of your most precious business assets – your people!

In the first part of this chapter, you will learn about the amazing power of compliments and how to effectively give them. In the second

Recognition is so easy to do and so inexpensive to distribute that there is simply no excuse for not doing it.
- Rosabeth Moss Kanter, author and management consultant, from *1001 Ways to Reward Employees*

The sweetest of all sounds is praise.
- Xenophon

part of this chapter, you will learn how to recognize your team on a regular basis.

Compliments

I agree with Dr. Marianne Kehoe of Geneva, Illinois, who says, "The most effective reward is a daily 'thank you' from the doctor for attentive staff." You can be the most intelligent and technically proficient professional in the world, but that isn't the most important thing to your staff. As Zig Ziglar says, "People don't care how much you know until they know how much you care – about them."

Here's what John Ball, service training manager, American Honda Motor Company, says about compliments. "I try to remember that people – good, intelligent, capable people – may actually need day-to-day praise and thanks for the job they do. I try to remember to get up out of my chair, turn off my computer, go sit or stand next to them and see what they're doing, ask about their challenges, find out if they need additional help, offer that help, if possible, and most of all, tell them that what they are doing is important – to me, to the company and to our clients."

In a second, you will learn the Five Steps to an Effective Compliment. Before we do that, let's look at five praising styles that don't work. They were identified by Brenda Barbour, Fortune Practice Management, San Diego, California.

I can live for two months on a good compliment.
- Mark Twain

Five Praising Styles That Don't Work

1. *Brush Off:* "You did a good job with that last patient. Would you go get our next patient now?"

2. *Comedian:* "Wow, I didn't think someone as small as you could take a stand with a big guy like that without being bulldozed over!"

3. *"What about me?:* "I'm glad you did so well on that project. I took myself off the project because I knew how important it was to you. It's great to see you accomplish what I planned."

4. *Flustered:* "Well, umm, you know, you really did, ahhhh a good job on collections this month. You, uh, really, you know, came through for us."

5. *"You did well, but . . . "*: "Shellie, you did a nice job going through the old charts, but in the future do it this way."

Giving an effective compliment, one that makes everyone feel good and encourages more of the complimented behavior is an art. Here is five-step blueprint you can use to give effective compliments today!

Five Steps to an Effective Compliment

1. Compliment the person as soon as possible after the behavior.

2. Begin the compliment with the person's name.

3. Compliment a *specific* action. It's important the person being complimented links the praise to a specific action taken. Now he or she knows exactly what to do again.

4. Explain *why* the action was important to you and the practice. This step adds an extra dose of meaning to the compliment.

5. End the compliment by asking a question to gain more information or "tie a bow" on the conversation by saying, "Keep up the great work!" or, "I really appreciate having you on our team!"

Following are two examples of effective compliments:

"Maria, you did a super job of calming down that child. That makes her mom feel more comfortable and it makes it easier for all of us. How did you learn to do that?"

"Michael, you did a great job with that veneer. The patient will be thrilled with the result. I really appreciate your dedication!"

You can compliment the staff members directly by communicating directly to them. You can also compliment them indirectly in two ways:

1. Tell the compliment to another team member or a patient. The people being complimented may or may not be present when you do this. If they aren't, you will be surprised the number of times the compliment "boomerangs" back to them.

2. Repeat a compliment about staff members you heard from patients. This will give the compliment new life!

They that value not praise will never do anything worthy of praise.
- Thomas Fuller

Good thoughts not delivered mean squat.
- Kenneth Blanchard, author and management consultant, from *1001 Ways to Reward Employees*

Do you single out individuals for public praise and recognition? Make people who work for you feel important? If you honor and serve them, they'll honor and serve you.
- Mary Kay Ash, founder, Mary Kay Cosmetics

Following are three examples of indirect compliments:

1. To a patient, "Mary did a wonderful job with your x-rays, Mrs. Logan. She's the best!"

2. To your entire staff, "Joan did a super job on collections this month. That's really going to boost everyone's bonus."

3. To your assistant, "Maria, Mr. Sanchez said you were the friendliest chairside assistant he has ever met. I appreciate everything you do for our office."

It's up to you to decide how to speak to your people.

Be a Storyteller

Another highly effective way to give a compliment and build an empowering office culture is to tell stories about office members who have done things you would like to see repeated. Great leaders in all fields are superb storytellers. Cultures that stand the test of time all have a frequently told collection of stories that convey what the culture is all about.

Stories are powerful for three reasons:

1. People get into stories. Watch people as they listen to an effective storyteller. It's almost as if they're hypnotized. They forget reality for a minute and become a participant in the story. When this happens, they experience the same emotions and learn the same lessons as the story characters.

2. Stories are indirect ways of conveying information. As an example, you can directly tell your staff you would like them to go the extra mile for your patients, or you can indirectly convey this message by telling an inspiring story about a staff member who went the extra mile for a patient. Which way do you think is most effective? You know the answer to that one.

3. Telling an inspiring story about a current staff member is a tremendous compliment to the person.

When You Give Compliments, Let People Know You Really Mean It

You have three tools of communication at your disposal when you give staff members compliments: your words, voice qualities and body language. Your words are what you're saying, your voice qualities are how you're saying it and your body language is the way you move your body as you say it.

Earlier in this chapter, you learned the words that work well when giving a compliment. However, words are your weakest tool of communication. They only account for 7 percent of the power of a compliment. More important are your voice qualities (38 percent) and body language (55 percent). So, when you give a compliment, put some emotion into it by "turning up the volume" in your voice qualities and body language.

Using Compliments to Reinforce New Behavior

Compliments are excellent ways of reinforcing a new action you would like to see in staff members. Use these three guidelines:

1. Don't wait for staff members to do the new action completely right before you compliment them. Compliment improvements. Here's an example, "Tanya, you're really getting better mixing that cement. Keep up the improvement!"

2. Compliment the person frequently at first. This is when they need the most reinforcement.

3. Decrease the frequency of the compliments as the action becomes natural.

Catherine Meek, president, Meek and Associates, says this about compliments, "In the twenty years of working with groups and interviewing thousands of employees in hundreds of companies, if I had to pick one thing that comes through to me loud and clear, it's that organizations do a lousy job of recognizing people's contributions. The number one thing employees say to me is, 'We don't even care about the money; if my boss would just say thank you, if he or she would just acknowledge that I exist. The only time I ever hear anything is when I screw up. I never hear when I do a good job.' Recognition programs are a very important element of your total compensation program."

There are dozens of things you could compliment your staff members on every day. It's up to you to turn the *could* into *will* on a daily basis!

Recognition

In Chapter 1, you learned that people act in ways that give them pleasure. In the first part of this chapter, you learned how to give staff members pleasure with compliments. Now, you will learn several ways to give even more pleasure by recognizing staff members for their achievements. Of course, you can recognize people one-on-one, but you can tremendously multiply the effect by "going public."

Five Ways to Multiply the Recognition Effect

1. *Include your office staff.* Following are seven ways you can do this:

Compensation is what you give people for doing the job they were hired to do. Recognition, on the other hand, celebrates an effort beyond the call of duty.
- Bob Nelson, author of *1001 Ways to Reward Employees*

    a. Hold a recognition ceremony in the office. Dr. Bill Howatt's office in Chapel Hill, North Carolina, does this with their "Bright Stuff Award." In their words, "We give the award to the person who comes to work and brightens everyone's day. The award is for any staff member, including the doctors, who focuses on the team and patients and brings joy to the office. This staff member puts happiness and joy first by role-modeling it daily. After a secret vote by the entire office, the award certificate is given once a month at one of our Thursday morning office huddles. The purpose of the Bright Stuff Award is to reward and celebrate the value of positive people in our office."

    b. "Tell all your staff members why they are a very important part of your team. Do it in front of the group at a staff meeting!" – Dr. Geeper Howard, Kings Mountain, North Carolina.

    c. "Establish a 'You Made My Day' Award. Buy a 'traveling award' (a stuffed animal toy, for example) that is given to a staff member who made someone's day. The winner can't keep the award for longer than a day. At the morning or evening huddle, the award is given to another staff member. Be sure to tell why the award is given."

    d. At the end of every staff meeting, encourage anyone to stand up and recognize another staff member for any reason.

e. Once a quarter, hold an "It's All About (staff member's name) Day." Gather interesting information, photos, childhood memorabilia, etc. from staff, family and friends. Hang a poster in the reception area with the heading "National Lisa Day!" Be sure to have a big picture of Lisa on the poster. Put some of the items you collected on or around the poster. At the end of the day, break out some sparkling apple cider and have everyone give a toast to Lisa. – Dr. Brad Shwidock, Stamford, Connecticut.

f. Collect patient letters praising the entire office and specific staff members. Make copies and distribute them to all your staff. If you hear a patient giving verbal praise, ask them to write it in a letter.

g. Create a "Bravo Board" and hang it in a place where the entire staff sees it frequently. Any staff member can write a Bravo Card to any other staff member and pin it to the Bravo Board.

2. *Include the staff member's family.* Write, call or tell face-to-face the staff member's spouse what a wonderful person he or she is married to. Let them know how much the staff member means to your practice. Conclude with, "I'm lucky to have (staff member's name) working with us!" Do the same with the staff member's parents.

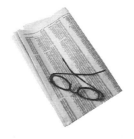

3. *Include your patients.* Put an article about a staff member in your patient newsletter. Tell your patients about their personal and professional lives, what the person means to your practice and some great things they've accomplished. You can do the same with a wall display in your reception area. – Dr. Paul Bass, Tullahoma, Tennessee.

We publish the accomplishments of our staff in the local newspapers. For example, 25 years of service to our local food bank or an award for making quilts. The staff member is honored, it creates great 'me too' with our current and future patients and the local newspapers love it. Everyone wins!
- Dr. Wes Teal, Loris, South Carolina

4. *Include your community.* Write a press release for your community or suburban newspaper that includes the achievements of a staff member. You may want to hire a professional writer if this isn't one of your strengths. In addition, when you speak at a community event, recognize your staff.

5. *Include your professional community.* Write a notice for a local or state professional newsletter that includes the achievements of your staff. In addition, when you speak at a professional meeting, recognize your staff.

Be Creative with Your Recognition

At the end of this chapter, I will give you a comprehensive list of ways to give compliments and recognition. Below is a short list of 12 ways you can be creative with your recognition:

1. *Give staff members a PASS IT ON Card from Argus Communications.* The PASS IT ON card has a butterfly and the saying, "Some people make the world more special just by being in it," on the front. On the back it reads PASS IT ON. When you give staff members the card, ask them, in the next 48 hours, to give it to another person who has done some little thing that makes a difference in their lives.

2. *Write a poem.* You may be a poet, and don't know it. In her wonderful book, *Care Packages*, Barbara Glanz tells a story of a way you can be creative with your recognition. Jim Munroe, an employee of a power company sends poems by e-mail to recognize his co-workers and to wish them happy birthday. He has received so much notoriety for doing this that he is now known as "The Workplace Poet!"

   Here is one of Jim's poems. It was sent to a person who does warehouse work:

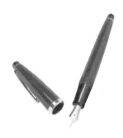

   You stock the shelves and that's not all,
   Shipping, receiving and telephone calls,
   Forms for this and forms for that,
   You even take care of old stray cats!
   So jump on that forklift and drive away,
   Have some cake and ice cream and a happy birthday!

3. *Write a simple and sincere letter of acknowledgement by hand.* The following will give you some content ideas. It's adapted from a chapter by Penny Reed in the book *FUNdamentals of Outstanding Dental Teams*, by Vicki McManus. Be sure to personalize your message as much as possible.

   Dear _____ ,

   You're such an important part of our team. I'd like to thank you for (pick one of the following):

   1. believing in my capabilities and me. Thank you for giving me unconditional support and complimenting my work.

2.   *your dedication. You've been with us for two years now, and I feel as if you're part of my family. Thanks for sticking with me during the good times and bad.*

3.   *your commitment to our patients. I've so much confidence in you and your abilities. It's nice to know I have you on the team to care for our patients.*

4.   *your caring spirit. Thank you for the compassion you show our patients and members of the team. You're a great listener and wonderful example.*

5.   *your honesty and commitment to open and supportive communication. I truly value your integrity.*

I admire your willingness to accept challenges and thoughtfulness to add value to our office. You're a valuable team member. Thank you for understanding we must have a profitable business in order to take care of our patients and ourselves.

Praise does wonders for the sense of hearing.
- Anonymous

I've really enjoyed the past two years, and I look forward to many more. Thanks for being on the team!

Your signature

4.   **Ask for their help.** Want to make your staff feel important? Ask for their help. Say, "I need some advice, can you spare a moment?" Turning to an employee for counsel sends a powerful message of trust and respect. Employees will scale mountains for doctors who demonstrate these qualities.

5.   **Are you "Out to lunch?"** One of the greatest gifts you can give people is the gift of your time. Once a month, take a staff member out to lunch. Just you and the team member. Use the opportunity to share praise and instill the positive values you want to see in your team. And most important, ask the person his or her ideas for improving the practice. This is another chance to show trust and respect.

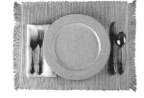

6.   **Assign a "Director of First Impressions."** Each month assign a Director of First Impressions. This person is responsible for coordinating everyone's efforts to ensure that your guests (read patients) feel cared for and welcomed. In addition, they are responsible for creating at least three new ways your office can show patients you care about

Recognition is something a manager should be doing all the time – it's a running dialogue with people. Compliments and recognition is not something that you turn off and on like a faucet. It's a habitual mind-set and course of action that can be crystallized in one sentence – I appreciate all the efforts of my staff, and I'm going to let them know I appreciate them by complimenting them and recognizing them whenever and where ever I can!
- Ron Zemke, senior editor of Training Magazine, from *1001 Ways to Reward Employees*

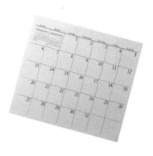

them. At the last staff meeting of the month, the Director shares his or her experience – what were the successes for the month, how did these successes improve the experience for everyone and their three improvements in patient care. At the conclusion of the meeting, assign a new Director of First Impressions for the following month.

Remember this: People are dying to feel good about themselves. When you give them the opportunity to do something nice for other people, you're presenting them with an opportunity to feel good about themselves.

7. *Use Recognition FUNdamentals from Baudville, Inc.* This is a terrific way to get started with your recognition and reward program. Recognition FUNdamentals contains Recognition Post-it® Notes, note cards, reward coupons, thank you cards and seals that you can use to let your team know you care.

8. *Leave a note of appreciation along with a small gift in the work areas of team members after they have left for the day.* It's a wonderful way for them to start their day.

9. *Use virtual postcards from iVillage.com.* These can be downloaded from the web at no cost. Select one of the available postcards (see Appendix A for more information).

10. *During the holidays write a short note to each staff member detailing the things you most value about working with that person during the year.*

11. *Use thank you cards from IntroKnocks.* Call for their catalog of unique recognition cards (see Appendix A for more information).

12. *On a calendar or in your contact management system, note the hiring date of all your staff members.* On that date, take them out to lunch, give them a unique gift described in Chapters 4 or 5 and let them know how much you appreciate another year of service.

13. *Use a calendar or your contact management system to alert yourself to special days such as staff birthdays and anniversaries.*

Here are four final thoughts about compliments and recognition:

1. *Never use respect as a reward*, i.e., "You do this, then I will respect you." Never withhold respect when you are upset with a staff mem-

ber, i.e., "You just did something I don't like. Now I don't respect you." Respect should always be present. It is unconditional.

2. *Use a 5:1 ratio for praise and correction.* Strive to praise staff members five times for every time you correct them. There are times when your staff does things that need to be brought to their attention and corrected. If you have praised them with the 5:1 ratio, they will accept your correction much better than if you never or rarely praise them.

3. *The foundation of praise is your attitude.* This chapter is loaded with dozens of ways you can praise your staff. Whether you use them or not, and how they're received will be determined by your attitude toward your people. Here's how three doctors put it:

"I have the best staff on earth. I don't shrink from anybody in telling this!" – Dr. Gayle Nelson, Sioux Falls, South Dakota.

"We continually recognize superior performance and acknowledge commitment beyond the call of duty. We reinforce those activities that allow the team to reach higher standards." – Dr. Jeff Priluck and Dr. Al Nordone, Dunwoody, Georgia.

I've got a question for you. Do you think that the staffs of Drs. Nelson, Priluck and Nordone sense their doctor's attitudes on a daily basis? And does this "knowing" of where they stand in their doctor's eyes influence their feelings toward the doctors and the amount of dedication and effort they put into the practice? I believe the answers to all these questions is a resounding, "Yes!" I hope you agree.

4. *You set the tone for the amount of praise given in your office.* Consider the message in the following story from the book *The Best of Bits & Pieces*:

A famous singer once contracted to appear at a Paris opera house. Ticket sales boomed, and the night of the concert found the house full and every ticket sold.

A feeling of anticipation and excitement was in the air as the house manager stepped out on the stage and announced, "Ladies and gentlemen, thank you for your enthusiastic support, but I have news that may be disappointing to some. An accident, not serious in nature but serious enough, will prevent the man you have come to hear from performing tonight." He went on to give the name of the

A man's inner nature is revealed by what he praises – a man is self-judged by what he says of others. Thus a man is judged by his standards, by what he considers the best. And you can't find a more crucial test. It reveals the soul.
- Hugo Black

understudy who would step into the role, but the crowd groaned and drowned it out. The excitement in the audience turned to bitter disappointment and frustration as the opera began.

The stand-in artist gave the performance everything he had. Throughout the evening, there had been nothing but an uneasy silence. Even at the end, no one applauded.

Then from the balcony, the thin voice of a little girl broke the silence. "Daddy," she called out, "I think you were wonderful!"

The crowd broke into thunderous applause.

In many ways, your dental office is the opera house. Your staff members are the understudy, and you are the little girl in the balcony. When you praise your teammates, after they have given their performances everything they have, the whole office will see and appreciate the person's effort and respond in kind.

A Comprehensive Compliment & Recognition List
As you go through this list, put a check mark in front of the ideas you're committed to using.

Compliments & Thank-Yous

○ Make a habit of saying, "Thank you," to individual staff members and your entire team.

○ Give a big, caring smile to your team members every day.

○ Compliment staff members face-to-face.

○ Leave a message of thanks on your staff members' voice mails.

○ Leave a message of thanks on your staff members' e-mails. This is especially nice to find at the beginning of the day.

○ Write compliments on Post-it® Notes. Put them in the people's work areas or hide them around the office.

○ Write compliments on purchased note cards. Be sure you have a supply of notes on hand at all times for everyone to use.

○ Hand-write thank you notes.

○ Write thank you notes on pay envelopes.

○ Print up your own cards with the word "Bravo" written on top. Encourage everyone in the office to use them.

○ Give birthday cards to your staff, their spouses and their children.

○ Present thank you cards in person, leave the card in the work area for the staff member to find or send the card to the person's home.

○ Compliment small improvements in behavior.

○ Compliment a staff member for a job well done in front of a patient.

○ Compliment a staff member by telling the compliment to other staff members.

○ Repeat compliments you hear about staff members.

○ Tell stories about the great things your staff has done.

○ Turn the volume up on your compliments by enhancing your voice qualities and body language.

○ Use compliments to reinforce new behavior you would like to see.

Recognition
○ Recognize your staff by congratulating them in person for an achievement.

Multiply the Recognition Effect – Include Your Office Staff
○ Create office awards and recognize staff members at your office meetings. Use a Bright Stuff Award.

○ Tell all staff members they are a very important part of the office team.

○ Create a traveling "You Made My Day" Award.

○ End every staff meeting with a round of recognitions.

○ Once a quarter hold an "It's All About (staff member's name) Day."

○ Collect letters praising the entire office and specific staff members. Make copies and distribute them to all your staff.

○ Create a Bravo Board and hang it in a place where the entire staff sees it frequently.

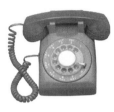

Multiply the Recognition Effect – Include the Staff Member's Family

○ Write, call and tell face-to-face the staff members' spouses what a wonderful person he or she is married to.

○ Write, call and tell face-to-face the staff members' parents what a wonderful son or daughter they have.

Multiply the Recognition Effect – Include Your Patients

○ Put an article about a staff member in your patient newsletter.

○ Recognize a staff member with a wall display in your reception area.

Multiply the Recognition Effect – Include Your Community

○ Write a press release for your community or suburban newspaper that includes an achievement by a staff member.

○ When you speak at a community meeting, recognize your staff.

○ Once a year take out an ad in the local newspaper thanking your staff for being the greatest!

Multiply the Recognition Effect – Include Your Professional Community

○ Write a notice for a local or state professional newsletter that includes the achievement by the staff member.

○ When you speak at a professional meeting, recognize your staff.

Be Creative with Your Recognition

○ Use PASS IT ON cards.

○ Write simple poems to your staff.

○ Hand write a simple and sincere letter of acknowledgement.

○ Ask for their help.

○ Take them out to lunch and solicit their suggestions for improving the office.

○ Assign a Director of First Impressions.

○ Use Recognition FUNdamentals from Baudville, Inc.

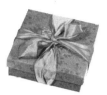

○ Leave a note of appreciation along with a small gift in the work area of a team member after he or she has left for the day.

○ Use virtual postcards from iVillage.com.

○ During the holidays write a short note to each staff member detailing the things you most value about working with that person during the year.

○ Buy and use thank you cards from IntroKnocks.

○ On a calendar or in your contact management system, note the hiring date of all your staff members. On that date, take them out to lunch, give them a unique gift described in Chapters 4 and 5 and let them know how much you appreciate another year of service.

○ Use a calendar or your contact management system to alert yourself to special days, such as staff birthdays and anniversaries.

Write your own compliments and recognition ideas below.

○ _____

○ _____

○ _____

○ _____

○ _____

○ _____

○ _____

A Recognition Fable

A frog asked two geese to take him south with them for the winter. At first the geese were reluctant, they didn't see how it could be done.

For some reason, there never seems to be enough recognition. After a brutal day, walk up to employees and say, 'You were great. I'm so glad about what you did today.' You'll be surprised how far a simple gesture will go.
- Robert Preziosi, president, Management Associates

Finally, the frog suggested the two geese hold a stick in their beaks, and he would hold on to it between them with his mouth. So off they went, flying southward over the countryside. It was an unusual sight. People looked up and admired their inspired teamwork. Someone shouted, "You are geniuses! Who was the clever one who thought of that wonderful way to travel?"

The frog couldn't resist. He opened his mouth and shouted back, "It was I," as he plummeted back to earth.

Don't be like the skydiving frog in the above fable. Give your team the credit for all the wonderful things your office accomplishes by complimenting and recognizing them whenever and where ever you can.

*Treat people as though
they were what they ought to be
and you help them become
what they are capable of being.*
- Goethe

Read the above quote again. Then answer these three questions:

1. What are the people in your practice capable of being?

2. How can you help them move in that direction with your compliments and recognition?

3. How would your practice be improved if these changes occurred?

In this chapter, you learned dozens of ways you can compliment and recognize your staff with little or no investment. Even though they don't cost much, it doesn't mean they aren't extremely powerful. In fact they are probably the most powerful kinds of recognition and rewards you can give! The rewards you learn in future chapters will seem hollow if you don't understand and use the things presented in this chapter.

Now it's time to move on to Chapter 3 – how you can reward your staff with . . . **Merchandise, Food and Clothing**.

3 | Merchandise, Food & Clothing

If you're like me, there are three things you want to accomplish in your dental practice:

1. Provide high quality care to hundreds of patients.

2. Create an environment where people enjoy their time in the office.

3. Create a practice where everyone does well financially.

An effective reward program accomplishes all three items listed above because it makes your staff feel appreciated. When they feel appreciated, they will enjoy themselves and want to provide high quality care for your patients. And finally, if some of your rewards are tied to a measure of performance, everyone will fare better financially.

As you learned in the last chapter, compliments and many types of recognition cost little or nothing. This chapter is a collection of over 350 merchandise, clothing and food ideas that have a monetary investment to them. As you did in the last chapter, put a check mark in front of the ideas that are possibilities for your staff. If appropriate, write the person's name next to the idea.

In his survey of 1,000 employees, Dr. Kenneth Kovach found that they value these 10 things the most:

1. Interesting work

2. Full appreciation for work done

3. Feeling included

4. Job security

Well-constructed recognition settings provide the single most important opportunity to parade and reinforce the specific kinds of new behavior one hopes others will emulate.
- Tom Peters, author and management consultant, from *1001 Ways to Reward Employees*

5. Good wages

6. Promotions and growth opportunities

7. Good working conditions

8. Personal loyalty to co-workers

9. Tactful disciplining

10. Empathetic help with personal problems

Does this list surprise you? Notice that the "intangible" things (1, 2, 3, 8, 9 and 10) outweigh the "tangible" things (4, 5, 6 and 7). I hope you see that an effective reward program can be a vital component of No. 2 - Full appreciation for work done, and No. 3 - Feeling included.

In this book, we're talking primarily about giving gifts to reward your staff. In reality, you can give gifts to:

1. Acknowledge	7. Thank
2. Praise	8. Recognize
3. Congratulate	9. Reward
4. Celebrate	10. Cheer
5. Motivate	11. Apologize
6. Promote	

Before you give a gift, have a specific purpose in mind. Then select a gift using the keys below as guidelines:

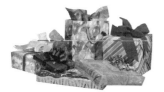

The Seven Keys to Selecting the Right Gift

The gift should meet most of the following criteria:

1. It is something the staff member desires.

2. It is useful – something the staff member uses frequently.

3. It has a high, perceived value in relationship to its cost.

4. It has lasting value.

5. It is a highly recognized and valued brand.

6. It is appropriate for the purpose given.

7. Its quality must reflect positively on your practice.

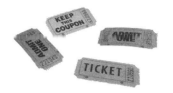

Here are some great ideas from other practices:

"I offer staff lunches, flowers, concert or theater tickets, restaurant gift certificates, continuing education trips to resorts or staff meetings/breaks at prestigious downtown Toronto hotel as rewards for ongoing staff support. These rewards could be for new patients referrals, working late or irregular hours, exceptional performance, a worthwhile suggestion that made our office more productive and profitable, or greater than average success at promoting unperformed dentistry." – Dr. David R. Jones, Cambridge, Ontario.

"I present an orchid to my assistants during Dental Assisting Week. I present the flowers to them at their favorite restaurant with thank you cards personally written by me." – Dr. Stephen Lawrence, Carlsbad, California.

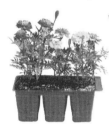

"One thing we do for our team is buy them a flowering plant for their desks about six times a year. It's nice to have blooming plants on each desk. Everyone appreciates it. For holidays, we buy a little memento for their desks filled with candy." – Alan and Sandy Richardson, Spokane, Washington.

"When we know of a special occasion in a staff member's life, we do something to surprise the person. We had a Lobster-Gram for our office manager's 25th wedding anniversary delivered to her home. We've also given theater tickets for a special day." – Dr. Martin Kolinski, St. Charles, Illinois.

"Give each staff member a crisp, new, $25, $50, or $100 bill rolled up and presented on the stem of a red rose." – Drs. Rick and David Howdy, Washington, North Carolina.

"Give each staff member a bottle of sparkling water or cider on the last working day of the month. If you choose, you can open one and celebrate with the team before going home." – Ed and Diann Crenshaw, Asheville, North Carolina.

"When the staff arrive at their work areas after the morning meeting, they find a bag full of 'hugs and kisses' with a hand-written thank you note from the doctor." – Ed and Diann Crenshaw, Asheville, North Carolina.

"Give each staff member a basket of foot-care products, including a foot soak! Present them at lunchtime." – Dr. Kani Nicolls, Asheville, North Carolina.

"Tie a balloon to each staff member's workstation that says, 'You're the Greatest,' or 'Good Job' or 'Yahoo.' Let them find the balloons after lunch." – Dr. Tom Tomlo, Hendersonville, North Carolina.

"Give out packages with aromatic energy boosters like soaps, candles and oils." – Dr. Kani Nicolls, Asheville, North Carolina.

"We give anniversary gifts at five and 10 years, which are presented at a staff luncheon. We give a watch or something equivalent at five years and a more expensive gift at 10 years. As examples, we've given a camcorder and a $700 landscape design gift certificate." – Dr. Martin Kolinski, St. Charles, Illinois.

Office Logo Merchandise Ideas

The merchandise listed below can be customized with your office name and logo. (See Appendix A for sources.)

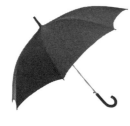

- ◯ t-shirts
- ◯ short-sleeve knit shirts
- ◯ sweat shirts
- ◯ jackets
- ◯ caps
- ◯ umbrellas
- ◯ mugs
- ◯ sports bottles
- ◯ gym bags
- ◯ carry-all bags
- ◯ stadium cushions
- ◯ golf accessories
- ◯ tennis accessories

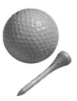

○ bowling accessories

○ coolers

○ coffee mugs

○ leather goods

○ pen and pencil sets

○ clocks

○ emery boards

○ business card magnets

○ paper weights

○ mouse pads

○ Post-it® Notes and pads

Write your ideas here:

○ _____

○ _____

○ _____

○ _____

○ _____

There is nothing more important than making certain each employee feels respected and valued.
- Robert Crandall, former CEO, American Airlines, from 1001 Ways to Reward Employees

There is one catalog every dental practice must order. The *Open Please* catalog contains dozens of great gifts – all with a dental theme. (See Appendix A.)

Just a reminder . . . are you putting check marks and names by the ideas that appeal to you?

Monogrammed Merchandise Ideas

Monogram these items with your staff members' initials. (See Appendix A for sources.)

- ○ towels
- ○ shirts
- ○ sweaters
- ○ shorts
- ○ athletic shoes
- ○ athletic shoe laces
- ○ athletic tote bags
- ○ crystal
- ○ stainless steel flatware
- ○ goblets
- ○ writing pens
- ○ gloves
- ○ golf balls
- ○ tennis balls

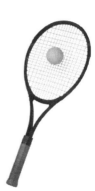

Write your ideas here:

- ○ _____
- ○ _____
- ○ _____
- ○ _____
- ○ _____

With so many ways to reward people, you may ask, 'How do I decide how to reward each person?' The answer is simple: Ask them.

- Michael LaBoeuf, author, from *1001 Ways to Reward Your Employees*

It's smart to vary the location where you present your rewards. Present gifts in your office. Have gifts sent to their homes. Present the gifts in special places such as restaurants or events.

Sports Team Merchandise Ideas

Many people love items featuring their favorite sports team. Most teams have official merchandise catalogs, stores and/or web sites. (Believe it or not, I could have made this list 10 times as long!)

○ t-shirts

○ short-sleeve knit shirts

○ sweat shirts

○ jackets

○ shorts

○ tank tops

○ jersey

○ bow ties

○ gym bags

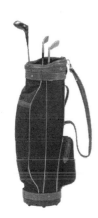

○ golf bags

○ golf putters

○ golf club covers

○ caps

○ socks

○ ties

○ purses

○ carry-all bags

○ coffee mugs

○ pasta

○ mini-helmets

*The heart of the giver makes
the gift dear and precious.*
- Martin Luther

- ○ pennants
- ○ poles and flags
- ○ wind chimes
- ○ bird houses
- ○ street signs
- ○ thermometers
- ○ magnets
- ○ jewelry
- ○ #1 foam fingers
- ○ balloons
- ○ leather goods
- ○ CDs
- ○ videos
- ○ cards
- ○ door mats
- ○ posters
- ○ pen and pencil sets
- ○ history books
- ○ belt buckles
- ○ shower curtains
- ○ robes
- ○ towel sets
- ○ tire covers
- ○ lamps
- ○ tableware
- ○ kids items

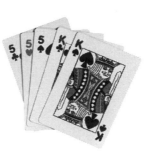

○ stadium chairs

○ stadium cushions

○ lamps

○ games

○ souvenir books

○ souvenir programs

○ autographed pictures, balls, programs and bats

○ watches

○ clocks

Write your ideas here:

○ _____

○ _____

○ _____

○ _____

○ _____

It's not the gift itself, but the idea behind it. It's nice to walk around the house and see an item and think, 'Oh, yeah, that's from 1984; I remember what I did for that one.' The memory the item gives you is so much better than money. Cash is here today, then gone tomorrow.

- Barion Mills, Jr., agency manager, State Farm Insurance, from 1001 Ways to Reward Employees

Presentation Is Everything

Your staff deserves their moment in the spotlight. You will want to show them with style just how grateful you are for their dedication and hard work. Following are some ideas:

1. Create excitement in the office by having a party for the recipient(s).

2. Give a short, heartfelt speech to let everyone know how you feel about the person, what the person did to deserve the award, and how that ties into the dream office you want to create. Remember, use your

words, voice qualities and body language to deliver a message that has meaning and impact.

3. Personally present the gift to the person.

4. Wrap the gift in nice paper with a ribbon and/or bow.

5. Always include a handwritten thank you note.

Electronics Ideas

Your favorite electronics store and catalogs, such as Sharper Image, are great sources for other ideas.

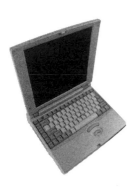

○ digital cameras

○ 35 mm cameras

○ video cameras

○ DVD players

○ compact disc players

○ VCRs

○ small color TVs for the kitchen

○ Sony Watch Man® portable TVs

○ laptop computers

○ Bose Wave® radios

○ coffee makers

○ waffle makers

○ electronic grills

○ air purifiers

○ water purifiers

○ cordless phones

○ electronic organizers

○ fax machines

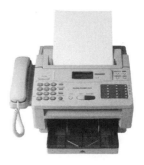

○ electronic musical keyboards

○ food processors

○ bread makers

○ microwave ovens

○ satellite dishes

○ power tools

○ educational or entertainment computer software

○ Internet access for one year

Write your ideas here:

○ _____

○ _____

○ _____

○ _____

○ _____

It's true that people can't be put in a neat box in a financial statement. You can't put a dollar figure on their net worth to the company. And you can't go to the bank and borrow against them. But people – not technology or fixed assets – are what determine the success or failure of any company.
- Roy Roberts, vice president of Personnel Administration, General Motors

Here are some more great ideas from other practices:

"We place long-stemmed roses on the keyboards of each terminal along with a gracious thank you note for the staff putting in extra time to convert our computer system!" – Dr. Brad Shwidock, Stamford, Connecticut.

"We really love random acts of kindness. This is exciting to the recipient and as satisfying and fun for the giver. We do random acts of kindness for our patients, our assistant, the amazing Lisa. As an example, Lisa and her husband went to the Catskills for a weekend. We sent a basket with champagne to their room. When they went to check out, they learned we had paid their entire bill. You can imagine the appreciation that she expressed to us." – Erica Silver, office manager for Dr. Peter Silver.

"If you have a mom who has put in extra time on a project, acknowledge her with a gift and give something to her kids – maybe video game rentals, movie rentals or amusement park passes." – Gary and NJ Miler, Columbia, South Carolina.

"We obtain the services of a personal shopper (i.e., Nordstrom) to perform a fashion makeover for each staff member. The staff can experience first-hand what it's like to be pampered while the shopper helps them select one complete outfit per staff member for them to take home." – Drs. Debra Gray King and Richard Creasman, Atlanta, Georgia.

"Get your staff involved in giving acknowledgements in a fun way. Initiate a Secret Pal program where any staff member can acknowledge, congratulate, celebrate, motivate, thank or cheer up another person. The program can be funded by your office. This adds another layer to your recognition and reward program." – Gary and NJ Miler, Columbia, South Carolina.

"One thing our team likes is the little party gifts they receive when we have them over for a dinner at Christmas or in the spring. In the spring, we decorate the patio with pretty potted flowering plants. At the end of the evening, each team member takes one of the plants home. We do the same thing at Christmas time with unique little candles and holders and flowering plants." – Dr. Reid Clark, Greensboro, North Carolina.

Just a reminder ... are you putting check marks and names by the ideas that appeal to you?

Other Reward Ideas
(See Appendix A for the sources of these specialty items.)

○ any item from the Tiffany catalog

○ any item from the Disney Store

○ any item from the Warner Brothers Store

○ Norman Rockwell calendars during the holiday season

○ work area items such as pens, organizers, small plants or holiday decorations

○ inspirational wall hangings, pictures or picture frames

○ small plants

○ balloons with messages on them

○ balloon bouquet with singing telegram

○ flowers for Valentines Day

○ flowers for birthdays

○ flowers for anniversaries

○ flowers with a "Thanks a Bunch" card

○ flowers for no reason at all

○ wall calendars

○ page-a-day calendars

○ auto accessories

○ items for their hobby

○ one red rose for each year of employment on their "anniversary"

○ items for the table – dinnerware, flatware, vases, glassware

○ picture of a scene you know they would enjoy

○ unique writing instruments

○ fiction books by their favorite authors

○ nonfiction books by their favorite authors

○ an autographed book by their favorite author

○ biographies and autobiographies of people they admire

○ cookbooks

○ journals and diaries

A surprise, no matter how small, is always welcome.
- Dr. Marianne Kehoe, Geneva, Illinois

○ travel log books

○ customized books or calendars

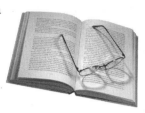

Books make fantastic gifts. Everybody has a favorite type of book or favorite author, so it's easy to give a uniquely desired gift. After you read a good book, pass it on to a staff member with a note that says, "I really enjoyed this book. I thought you would enjoy it as well."

You can also buy a best-selling book on customer service for each staff member. Have them read one chapter a week and discuss the chapter at your weekly team meeting.

○ note cards with prestamped envelopes

○ a subscription to their favorite magazine

○ photo albums

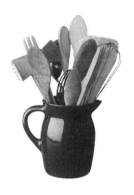

○ cookware

○ knives

○ kitchen gadgets

○ unusual dinnerware, linens, etc. – summer patterns, for example

○ educational or inspirational audiotapes, videotapes or CDs

○ twelve long-stemmed, chocolate roses with silk leaves in a gift box

○ watches

○ a watch that you can add a diamond to for each year of employment

○ clocks

○ binoculars

○ a newspaper published on the day they were born

○ instructional videos for golf, tennis, cooking, home improvement, etc.

○ travel videos

○ towels

○ necklaces

○ earrings

○ pins

○ cultured pearls

○ bracelets

○ charms

○ pendants

○ pen and pencil sets

○ crystal

○ porcelain

○ silverware

○ stainless steel

○ silver plate gifts

○ serving trays

○ unusual lights

○ sculptures

○ candles

○ picture frames

○ crystal perfume bottles

○ additional items for their collections (Beanie Babies®, Boyd's Bears®, Precious Moments®, Dickens Village®, etc.)

○ greeting cards containing taped messages for special occasions

○ garden tools

○ garden seeds and bulbs

○ luggage

○ telescopes

Looking for unique gifts?
Check out Appendix A for a complete list of resources.

❍ furniture

❍ antiques

❍ home exercise equipment

❍ gourmet gardens in boxes

❍ ornaments for the Christmas tree

❍ holiday season decorations for their homes

❍ gourmet coffee or tea

❍ outdoor flags and banners

❍ a bright red dinner plate for a special person

❍ outdoor or camping equipment

❍ patio or barbecue equipment

❍ pool accessories

The way we see it, spending $1 on something clever and unique is better than spending $50 on something ordinary and forgettable.
- Richard File, partner, Amrigon, from *1001 Ways to Reward Employees*

Write your ideas here:

❍ _____

❍ _____

❍ _____

❍ _____

❍ _____

Gift Investment Amounts

According to a recent survey of corporations done by the Promotional Products Association (percentages add up to more than 100 percent because people were purchasing gifts in more than one price range):

- **27 percent** of the respondents were purchasing gifts in the $1 to $5 range

- **32 percent** of the respondents were purchasing gifts in the $6 to $10 range

- **40 percent** of the respondents were purchasing gifts in the $11 to $25 range

- **38 percent** of the respondents were purchasing gifts in the $26 to $50 range

- **23 percent** of the respondents were purchasing gifts in the $51 to $100 range

- **17 percent** of the respondents were purchasing gifts in the over $100 range

Food

Food is always a welcomed gift . . . the healthier the better (See Appendix A for sources.) There is one challenge with a food gift – when they eat it, it's gone!

> "Add healthy food to your staff's benefit plan by giving them an "Employee Saver Card" obtained from local restaurants. The card entitles the bearer to 15 percent off, and they are reusable. It's a great idea for all of the staff. It helps them with the cost of lunch and saves them time since they don't have to make their lunch in the morning!"
> – Dr. Stephen Lawrence, Carlsbad, California.

Just a reminder . . . are you putting check marks and names by the ideas that appeal to you?

Food Reward Ideas

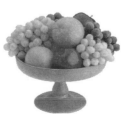

○ fresh fruit baskets

○ fresh Georgia peaches for the "peach" of your practice

○ batch of fresh chocolate chip cookies

○ fillet mignon steaks

○ fresh Maine lobsters

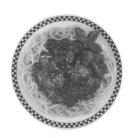

- fresh oysters for the "pearl" of your practice
- gift packed ham, turkey, Canadian bacon, pork chops or baby back ribs
- pizza to take home for dinner
- pasta dinners in pasta pots they can keep
- complete chicken dinners to take home for dinner
- catered dinners from ethnic restaurants in their homes
- five-foot sub sandwiches
- catered breakfast from the best breakfast place in town for the entire office
- catered breakfasts for staff members in their homes – they can be two hours "late" that day.
- romantic dinner for two at a four-star restaurant
- bottle of champagne or wine
- gourmet popcorn or nuts
- gourmet coffees
- fresh bagels delivered to the office once a month
- a different specialty bread every month for every staff member
- a special dish you make just for them
- fortune cookies with personalized messages
- cookie bouquets
- personalized cakes
- sparkling cider
- exotic teas
- truffles
- seasonal chocolates
- Jelly Bellies®

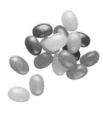

Write your ideas here:

○ _____

○ _____

○ _____

○ _____

○ _____

Remember the happy times (birthdays, anniversaries, graduations, births) and the not-so-happy times (deaths of family members, sicknesses).

Set up a calendar event file to alert you to special staff events, birthdays, anniversaries, etc.

Clothing Ideas

You can buy the gift yourself; have the person choose from a catalog; or give a gift certificate. The gift will be more special if it's something they would never buy for themselves. They will think of you every time they wear it. Suggested items include:

○ hats

○ sweaters

○ shirts

○ scarves

○ accessories

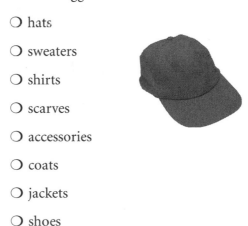

○ coats

○ jackets

○ shoes

○ dresses

○ aprons

○ pants

○ exercise clothing

○ clothing for a favorite sport

Write your ideas here:

○ _____

○ _____

○ _____

○ _____

○ _____

Sometimes a gift and/or a birthday card to a family member (parent, spouse, child, brother, sister, pet) can have even more impact than a gift to the staff member.

Get more bang for your buck by using your patients as vendors for some of your recognitions and rewards. Do you have any patients who own restaurants, bakeries, flower shops, or provide a service such as massage or manicures? Include them in the fun!

In this chapter, you learned over 320 ways to reward your staff with merchandise, food and clothing. I don't ever want to hear you say, "I just don't know what to get people." You've just put check marks in front of numerous ideas. Now you need to take action on your ideas in the days, weeks and months ahead. Speaking of taking action – you will want to move to Chapter 4 right now. Be prepared to learn how to use **Money and Gift Certificates**.

4 | Money & Gift Certificates

In the last chapter, you learned how to use merchandise, food and clothing in your office reward program. In this chapter, you will add two additional tools to your reward toolbox – money and gift certificates.

Money is like closet space. You use up as much as you have.
- Ray Michel

Money

I thought this would be one of the easiest chapters to write. After all, common wisdom says that, in a work situation, people are motivated most by money. Remember the employee study from Chapter 1. Managers ranked good wages as No. 1 on a list of ten factors employees desire in a job. In reality, it's been one of the hardest chapters to write. Money is important, but it's not all that its cracked up to be. Consider the following:

1. Unlike their managers who rated money No. 1, employees rated it No. 5 on the list of ten factors. The employees rated "full appreciation of work done" as No. 1.

2. Money is effective in attracting and keeping good people, but it doesn't motivate them to do their best work. Money will influence your people to go halfway up the mountain. It won't inspire them to reach the mountaintop.

3. Money can be exciting when you get it, but it has no lasting value.

4. Money is needed, but it's not special. It tends to be spent on bills and "stuff."

5. Money is desired, but it tends to become an expected reward. A salary

is a good example of this. This is why a raise in salary is a poor way to motivate long-term behavior.

So if money isn't what your staff desire most, what is it? In my experience of working with hundreds of organizations and ten of thousands of people, I believe it boils down to four factors:

1. *Being part of an organization that has a purpose that is more than just making money.* All professional practices should fall into the category. As the leader, you need to live this purpose in word and deed.

2. *Being fully appreciated and respected.* As the leader, you need to practice the concepts presented in this book first – especially the ones presented in Chapter 2.

3. *Being a vital part of the organization.* Being an active participant in decision making and sharing in the emotional and financial rewards of the practice. As the leader, you need to create a synergistic team that becomes more than the sum of its parts.

4. *Having a challenging job that stimulates learning and growth.* As the leader, you need to make sure that everybody on your team has the opportunity to expand their boundaries.

So if money won't inspire your people to do their best work, to get them to the mountaintop, what will it do? Good question.

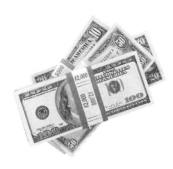

1. Money can be given in doses as part of a long-term reward program. Salaries are an example of this.

2. Money can be used as an incentive to inspire short-term behavior. As an example, "If we have 25 new patient exams in the month of September, everyone gets a $100 bonus. What are some things we can do to make that happen?"

3. Money can spark creative thinking. See the **Use Money to Reward Creative Improvement** section on the next page.

Use Money as an Incentive for Achieving a Short-Term Performance Goal

You can use monetary awards as an incentive for achieving a performance goal such as production, number of new patients, net profit and/or reduction in expenses for a specified time period. Here are the keys you will want to remember:

1. Set a realistic, achievable and measurable goal.

2. Clearly communicate what the monetary incentive will be.

3. Limit the time period to no more than three months.

4. Keep the rules simple.

5. Link the incentive directly to office or area performance.

6. Involve as many people as possible.

7. Give the incentive promptly.

Use Money to Reward Creative Improvement Ideas

The quality level of your office is never staying the same – it's either getting a little bit worse every day, or it's getting a little bit better every day. If you're not constantly focusing on getting better, guess which way your practice is going? To create your dream practice, you must make plussing a way of life in your office. Walt Disney defined plussing as the gradual improvement of your business every single day. It's the little things, performed over and over during the year that make a big difference at the end of the year. The difference between excellence and mediocrity can often be found in the little things.

Here's a great example of plussing from the world of sports. At the end of the year, the difference between the No. 1 money winner on the men's professional golf tour and those in the middle of the pack is 1.5 strokes per round – about a 2 percent difference!

I strongly recommend the book *Walt Disney – An American Original,* by Bob Thomas. In it, Thomas relates, "During his visits to Disneyland, Walt was always plussing – looking for ways to improve the appearance of Disneyland and provide more pleasure for the guests. He would study an area and tell his staff, 'Let's get a better show for the guests: what can we do to give this place more interest?'"

One of the reasons Toyota makes great cars is that they know the value of plussing. In 1984, Toyota received 2,150,000 suggestions from its employees for improvements in the way the company makes cars and does business. Then, Toyota implemented an astonishing 96 percent of them!

Give a percentage of the profit for the first 60 days that a new income center is established, i.e. bleaching, Oxyfresh, etc.
- Dr. Paul Bass, Tullahoma, Tennessee

There's an old business slogan that says, "That which gets measured and rewarded, gets done." If constant improvement of your practice is important to you, you must make improvement a priority by constantly collecting great ideas from all of your staff, rewarding them for their ideas and then taking action on most of the ideas.

Here is a nine-step plan you can use to make plussing a way of life in your dental office:

1. In written and verbal form, communicate to your team that the next staff meeting is going to focus on ideas that will improve the practice in a certain area. Word the communication like this: "Our next staff meeting is going to focus on (pick one of the areas below):

    ○ how we can improve the quality of our existing services
    ○ how we can enjoyably increase production
    ○ how we can enjoyably increase collections
    ○ how we can attract more quality patients to our practice
    ○ how we can decrease expenses without affecting quality
    ○ how we can enjoyably get more done in the same or less time
    ○ how we can bring more enjoyment to our time in the office

    Please bring your best ideas. The ideas can be big ones or small ones. The ideas can be related to your area or someone else's area. The ideas can focus on new or existing services we provide. Any idea that improves our office in this area is fine. Everyone is expected to participate. You will be rewarded with $5 cash for each idea you share. Up to three ideas per person, please."

2. At the meeting, one at a time, go around the room and ask people their ideas. Do not debate, judge or evaluate the ideas. Announce this ahead of time. Appoint a person to write down all ideas. You may need to clarify an idea with its creator.

3. Immediately give the person the appropriate number of $5 bills and move on to the next person. If a person has no ideas, say nothing and move on. When you have asked the entire group, thank them and explain what's going to happen with their ideas. See Step Four.

4. The night of the meeting, sit down with all of the ideas and put them into four categories:

a. the ideas that are workable and can be acted on without anyone else's input

b. the ideas that seem good and need someone else's input – the idea's originator or someone directly affected by the idea

c. the ideas that seem workable, but because of time or money, need to be delayed

d. the ideas that you don't believe will work at this time

5. Inform the idea's originator of the status of their ideas the next day. This can be done in writing. Be sure to thank them for each idea.

6. With all the workable ideas above, assign one or more persons to put the ideas into action. Often, the person most motivated to put an idea in action and see it succeed is the person who recommended it. With all ideas that need more input, hold a short meeting with the appropriate people, and assign someone to put the ideas into action. Be sure to agree on deadlines.

7. Create a system to measure and evaluate the idea's success. Refine the idea if necessary.

8. At the next staff meeting, have the responsible people give a short report of their progress including the positive results they've achieved.

9. Introduce a new area of plussing focus for your next staff meeting.

You might be thinking to yourself, "Well, my staff should be doing this anyway. Why should I pay them extra for something they should be doing in the first place?" That's a valid question. In reality, some of their ideas would have been brought to your attention, and I know you will find that a lot more would not have been identified. You can stimulate the imagination of your staff. The plussing process above sensitizes people to look for improvements everywhere. They will see things they hadn't seen before. Do the nine-step plussing process, and you will be amazed with the results.

Finding that better way is rewarded at GE.
- Jack Welch, chairman, General Electric

The nine-step plussing process outlined above is a great way to jump-start the creative idea process. Once it has gained momentum, you can maintain it with a creative compensation process with a built-in reward system like the one described in Chapter 7.

Be Careful to Reward the Behavior You Desire

There once was a man with a dog named Fred. One day, Fred brought home a live bird in his mouth. His master commanded Fred to drop the bird. After Fred did as he was instructed, his master petted him and gave him a treat. The next day Fred brought home two birds in his mouth.

At one time, Pizza Hut rewarded their drivers for delivering pizza in twenty minutes or less. After a series of lawsuits, Pizza Hut realized they were also rewarding the drivers for speeding and reckless driving.

Don't make similar mistakes like Fred's master and Pizza Hut. Always have a clearly defined purpose for rewarding your staff. The reward can be:

1. **A ritual** - their paychecks, holiday season bonuses, birthday gifts. These are the rewards most offices use. There's nothing wrong with them, but because they are expected, they have the least impact.

2. **"Out-of-the-Blue"** - gifts given just because you appreciate and respect your people. Out-of-the-Blue rewards increase the staff members' appreciation and respect for you.

3. **An Unanticipated Reward** - bouquets of flowers after a tough day or unexpected monetary bonuses after a great month. Unanticipated rewards reinforce desired behavior and increase the likelihood that the behavior will occur again in the future.

4. **An Incentive** - an extra day off during the holiday season when you increase production 10 percent during November or a trip to Orlando when you hit a net profit goal. Incentive rewards increase the likelihood of your staff changing their behavior so you achieve your desired outcomes.

A well-planned reward program includes all four types of rewards listed above. Sincerity, variety and consistency are the keys to an effective plan. In Chapter 9, you will use all the information in this book to construct your reward program.

Ways Other Offices Use Money as a Reward

"We give monetary rewards, to employees who go above and beyond. Although the tax advantages may not be there with this type of reward, the benefits are worth it. The dollar amount is usually in the $50 - $100 range." – Dr. Martin Kolinski, St. Charles, Illinois.

"In an effort to make chart audits more fun, we've had offices hide money and gift certificates in the charts to make the process a treasure hunt." – Gary and NJ Miler, Columbia, South Carolina.

"We present staff members with a money bag full of Susan B. Anthony silver dollars – 25 to 50 per bag." – Ed and Diane Crenshaw, Asheville, North Carolina.

"When one of our two offices was sold, Dr. Kolinski very generously gave Maria, our office manager, and me a bonus. This was to say "thank you" for all the years of hard work in that office, as well as to thank us for the effort that went into the sale of the practice." – Dr. Martin Kolinski staff member, St. Charles, Illinois.

"At staff meetings, each staff member is given a $5 bill to award to another in recognition of "above and beyond" behavior. This encourages all of us to catch other staff members doing something good and keeps us aware of how important it is to look for opportunities to help. Praise from peers feels great!" – Dr. Terri Brummitt, San Jose, California, from FUNdamentals of Outstanding Dental Teams.

"Create a financial freedom game plan for your staff. Their tendency will always be to want immediate gratification. Later, they will be glad you helped them put the plan in place. My personal staff has reached that point, and it's a neat feeling to know how appreciative they are. You can also start ROTH IRAs for the staff's children. Put in $100 a year and demonstrate to the staff how the money will be in the retirement account at age 65 with various interest rates." – Dr. Paul Bass, Tullahoma, Tennessee.

"In the months that we show higher than average production and collections, we issue payroll bonuses - usually $100 - 200. This shows that we recognize and appreciate that everyone worked a little harder than normal." – Dr. Martin Kolinski, St. Charles, Illinois.

More Creative Ways to Give Your Staff Money as a Reward

1. Provide free or reduced cost professional care to the staff and/or their family.

2. Give a $500 bonus when they have a baby.

3. Donate money to their favorite charity.

4. Pay a portion of their mortgage for a month around the holiday season.

5. Pay for a portion of their childcare for the summer.

6. Pay for their child's tutoring if you hear the child is having trouble with a certain subject at school.

7. Pay for their uniform cleaning.

8. Give silver dollars.

9. Give gold coins.

10. Give a rare coin with a note saying, "This coin is as rare as you are."

11. Hide a $20 bill in their work area with a note saying, "Have a little extra fun this weekend!"

12. Give $100 per quarter for perfect attendance.

13. Give shares of an industry-related stock.

14. Give savings bonds.

Everyone works smarter when there is something in it for them. -Michael LaBoeuf, author, The Greatest Management Principle in the World, from *1001 Ways to Reward Employees*

Gift Certificates

Gift certificates are an excellent way to put money into people's pockets. They can direct people to spend money on things not normally purchased.

"We give membership cards to all of our staff to places like Costco and Sam's Club. It saves the employees a lot of money all year long." – Dr. Stephen Lawrence, Carlsbad, California.

Creative Ways To Give Your Staff Gift Certificates
Check the ideas that appeal to you.

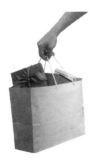

○ gift certificates from their favorite music, book or clothing stores

○ gift certificates from their favorite restaurants or the best restaurant in town – one they would say is "too expensive"

○ gift certificates from their favorite mall or discount stores

○ gift certificates for home cleaning, chimney sweeping, yard maintenance or home repairs

○ gift certificates for golf, tennis, dance or bowling lessons

○ gift certificates for scuba or sky diving

○ gift certificates for a rafting adventure

○ gift certificates for a glider, biplane or hot air balloon ride

○ gift certificates for a harbor or ocean cruise

○ gift certificates for weekend convertible or sports car rental

○ gift certificates for craft, pottery or art lessons

○ gift certificates for massages, facials, health clubs or day spas

○ gift certificates for a weekend get-away at a bed-and-breakfast or hotel

○ gift certificates for cosmetic surgery

○ gift certificates for pet grooming or kennel services

○ gift certificates for child care or kid's camp

○ gift certificates for family portraits

○ movie passes

○ raffle tickets

○ lottery tickets

○ tickets to plays, amusement parks, concerts, cultural events, comedy clubs or sporting events

○ front row tickets to events

○ entertainment coupon books

Treasure Chest

Keep a drawer in your desk full of all-occasion cards, gift certificates and small gifts for those times when you need to recognize a person for going above-and-beyond the call of duty.

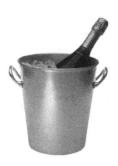

Combine Activities to Create "The Perfect Day"

On my wife's birthday a few years ago, I created a perfect day for her. She started at a beauty shop where she received a facial, manicure and pedicure. The shop owner then gave her directions to her favorite restaurant where she had her favorite lunch, which had already been paid for. The restaurant gave her directions to a location where she received a massage. The masseuse gave her directions to one of her favorite stores where a gift certificate was waiting for her to use. The storeowner gave her directions to a flower shop where a bouquet of her favorite flowers was waiting. The flower shop owner instructed her to go home where I was waiting for her with some champagne. I'll stop the story here to preserve the G rating of this book.

Add Some "Pop" to Your Gift Certificate Giving

Inflate some balloons and insert slips of paper that entitle the "popper" to any of the ideas listed in this chapter. During a staff meeting, recognize a staff member who has demonstrated exceptional patient service that month. Be sure to tell everyone what the person did and the result it created for the patient. The team member selects a balloon and pops it to reveal a special gift of thanks.

Take a second now to review this chapter. What ideas has it stimulated? What actions are you committed to taking in your practice? Write your answers in the space below.

1.

2.

3.

4.

5.

No social system will bring us happiness, health and prosperity unless it is inspired by something greater than materialism.
- Clement Attlee

The quote above applies to your office social system too. The material rewards presented in this book will fall flat on their faces if you don't move beyond their materialism. You must add healthy and frequent doses of personal caring and appreciation for your staff. When you add this to an office purpose that enhances your patients' lives, you will have the happiness, health and prosperity you all desire!

Your reward toolbox is getting fuller by the minute. In Chapter 2, you learned how to give compliments and use recognition. In Chapter 3, you learned to give merchandise, food and clothing wisely. In this chapter, you learned how the do's and don'ts of effectively giving money and gift certificates. Keep the momentum going. Turn to Chapter 5 right now and learn the "ins and outs" of . . . **Celebrations and Activities**.

5 | Celebrations & Activities

In the last chapter, you learned how to use money and gift certificates in your reward program. In this chapter, your creativity will truly come into play. You will learn how to have celebrations and activities that reward your staff for a job well done.

Before we move on, there's a topic that should be raised. Some dentists resist using rewards because they fear their staff will come to expect the rewards. They believe the rewards will lose their value with time, and/or there will be negative feelings created if the rewards are not given. This is a valid concern, and can be prevented from happening by following these four guidelines:

1. *Use a variety of rewards.* As an example, when you make your numbers in the first quarter, take the staff and their partners out to dinner at a nice restaurant. In the second quarter, give them a half-day off. In the third quarter, present each person a gift selected just for him or her. In the fourth quarter, have a "Ferris Buehler afternoon" where everyone goes out, has fun in their own unique way, and comes back at 4:30 to report what they did. The variety will add fun to your office and decrease the expectations that may come with repeatedly using the same reward.

When creating an incentive, managers should focus on results, not activity.
- George W. Walther, president, Tel Excell Companies, from 1001 Ways to Reward Your Employees

2. *Emphasize non-monetary rewards.* Studies have shown that, on a dollar-to-dollar basis, non-monetary rewards are more effective than monetary rewards. This book gives you over 500 ways you can reward your staff with non-monetary rewards.

3. *Link rewards to results.* When you link rewards to results, (exceed-

ing a collection goal), you make the success of the practice the primary focus. When you link rewards to employment (turkeys for everyone at Thanksgiving), you create an atmosphere of entitlement.

4. *Add emotion to each reward.* Be sure you give the reward with the emotions of love and gratitude wrapped around it. This will multiply the value of the reward and make you and the staff member feel great!

In the first half of this chapter, you will learn how to stage celebrations that make a difference. In the second half of this chapter, you will learn how to produce activities that instill a sense of team spirit.

Celebrations

All cultures that have stood the test of time have numerous celebrations. Celebrations are fun to attend, and they're beneficial to the culture for at least six reasons.

Six Benefits of Celebration

1. *Celebration gives you a sense of history.* A celebration today gives the entire team something to remember. It literally gives your team a sense of history and the positive experiences associated with it. Be sure to take pictures of all your celebrations and put them somewhere they can be viewed easily.

2. *Celebration builds relationships.* Celebrations allow people to get to know each other outside of their usual professional roles.

3. *Celebration helps your team envision the future.* Like a wedding, when you celebrate beginnings (a new staff member, a new operatory, a new year), you symbolize your commitment to the future.

4. *Celebration helps you recognize major milestones.* This reminds everyone that they are part of a winning team and reinforces the actions that led to the achievement.

5. *Celebration helps reduce stress and reenergizes people.* At the very least, celebrations give people a change of pace and allow them to recharge their batteries.

6. *Celebration creates enthusiasm, which nourishes the spirit.* The word

enthusiasm comes from the Greek words *en theos*, meaning God-like. That's a clue to the power of enthusiastic, fun-loving celebrations.

Outstanding celebrations don't just happen. Following are six guidelines to follow to ensure your celebrations produce the results you desire.

Six Guidelines for an Outstanding Celebration

1. *The celebration must be authentic.* Celebrations must spring from your genuine appreciation for your staff. You must believe that your practice's success is achieved through the efforts of the entire team. One definition of the word celebrate is "to praise."

2. *The celebration must include as many people as possible in the planning.* If you're not good at or don't enjoy planning celebrations, I can almost guarantee there is one or more of your staff who would love to do it. Tap into their creativity and enthusiasm. Then sit back and enjoy the ride.

3. *The celebration must be fun.* Link joy and fun to your celebrations so that people will want to join in and contribute in the future.

4. *The celebration must involve all of the senses.* When you plan celebrations, involve the senses of sight (decorations), hearing (music), touch (respectful hugs), taste (healthy foods) and smell (healthy foods), you indelibly imprint the experience on your staff's nervous systems.

5. *The celebration must be seen as an investment.* When people are celebrated (praised), they have higher job satisfaction, morale, productivity and esprit de corps. These emotions have direct, bottom-line benefits.

6. *The celebration must be cost-effective.* Spending a lot of money is not a necessary ingredient for an effective celebration. The interaction of the people is the main ingredient.

"One day every summer we have an in-office beach party complete with beachwear and music. We include our patients in the fun!" – Dr. Marshall Fields, Columbia, South Carolina.

"Many times, for no reason at all, or if we have a highly productive day, someone on the team will mention that this would be a great

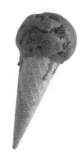

day for a celebration. We may bring in ice cream, cake and drinks, or we might go out for appetizers. It's a great way to say, "Thank you for working so hard!" – Dr. Michael Koczarski, Woodenville, Washingon.

"We celebrate employees' birthdays. The whole team is treated to a special birthday lunch with birthday cake. We love our annual holiday party. The team goes out to dinner and has "fun and games" with their spouses or dates." – Dr. Wes Teal, Loris, South Carolina.

Some Things You Can Celebrate

Celebrate in or out of the office. Check the ones that appeal to you.

○ birthdays

○ engagements

○ weddings

○ work anniversaries - one rose for every year of service

○ wedding anniversaries

○ graduations, achievements and promotions

○ staff members joining or leaving the team

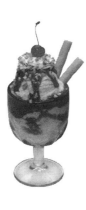

○ office goals achieved - for example, celebrate the end-of-the-month performance with an ice cream party complete with the makings for world-class sundaes or banana splits. Include ice cream, toppings, bananas, cherries and whipped cream

○ New Year's - everyone tells their most important New Year's resolution. Everyone else commits to helping them achieve it

○ Valentines Day - everyone receives a "You Are Loved" pin

○ St. Patrick's Day - green-colored popcorn in bags for all the patients and staff

○ Cinco de Mayo (Mexican Independence Day) - tacos, burritos, chips and salsa for everybody

○ Independence Day - lowfat yogurt and red, white and blue balloons

○ Halloween - wear costumes like the Southwest Airlines employees

○ Thanksgiving - each staff member brings their favorite dish for a potluck lunch

○ kids day at the office - kids come to see what mom and dad really do

○ Elvis's birthday - grilled bacon, peanut butter and banana sandwiches for lunch, Elvis Music on the sound system, etc.

○ 50's day - 50's music and dress

○ Hawaiian Shirt Gonzo Friday - wild shirts and attitudes

○ Salmon-Chanted Evening - go out for a fish dinner with staff and their families

○ bad socks day - include your patients on any day when they can join in on the fun

○ crazy hat day

○ April is National Humor Month - every day in April, one staff member tells a joke and brings a cartoon for the bulletin board

○ November is National Peanut Butter Month - every day someone brings a creative peanut butter treat for the office

○ How about celebrations for these days?

- January 27 - National Popcorn Day
- March 22 - National Goof Off Day
- June 12 - National Hug Day
- July 3 - Dog Days of Summer begins
- August 12 - Bad Poetry Day
- October 12 - Moment of Frustration Scream Day

○ Any other crazy day you can think of

"Postpone the traditional December holiday celebrations until late January. This reduces holiday stress and gives the staff something to look forward to during the winter months. Make the time spent together really fun with gag gifts, photos of events during the year and special awards." – Dr. Robert Boe, Atlanta, Georgia.

"We have celebrated exceeding our annual goals by giving each staff member an all-inclusive Caribbean weekend get-a-way for two taken at a time of their choice." – Dr. Debra Gray King and Richard Creasman, Atlanta, Georgia.

"You don't always need the whole team to celebrate. Small successes can be celebrated by one or two team members and then shared with the entire team later. Some celebrations can be spontaneous – a group cheer followed by high-fives. When you're surprised by results or events, celebrate!" – Gary and NJ Miler, Columbia, South Carolina.

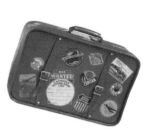

OOPS. Let's Party

Be sure to celebrate your well-intentioned mistakes as well. Mistakes are a prerequisite for growth. It signals that your team is leaving its comfort zone and moving to the next level. Remember, as an airplane rises to the next level, it encounters turbulence, and the ride is often a bumpy one. It's only after the plane has reached its cruising attitude that the "fasten seat belt" sign is turned off.

Activities

Like celebrations, well-planned activities are an important part of your recognition and reward program and just plain fun. Southwest Airlines has made having fun a way of business. If you've ever flown Southwest, you know what I mean. I was on a Southwest Airlines flight from San Diego to Phoenix recently. The man in front of me opened the overhead compartment door to put his briefcase in. As he did, a flight attendant stuck her head out and shouted, "BOOOOO!" The whole plane cracked up. We proceeded to have a wonderful trip over to Phoenix.

What isn't widely known is that having fun is good business. Just ask Southwest Airlines. In addition to having the funniest people in the business, Southwest Airlines:

- gets its planes in and out of terminals in about half the time of most airlines

- is the No. 1 airline in on-time performance and baggage handling

Every human being either adds to or subtracts from the happiness of those with whom he or she comes into contact.
- Anonymous

Humor is counterbalance. Laughter need not be cut out of anything, since it improves everything.
- James Thurber

- has less than half the complaints per passenger than the No. 2 airline on the list

- has never had a serious accident or fatality in 27 years of flying.

Like Southwest Airlines, I believe having more fun will provide your office with at least four valuable benefits.

Four Benefits of Fun

1. *Your office will be more productive.* Southwest Airlines has the smallest number of employees per aircraft and serves the most customers per employee. People who are having fun get more done.

2. *Your office will have lower absenteeism and turnover.* When your staff truly enjoys their time in the office, they will want to come to your office each day. They also will want to stay working with you, even though they could make a few more dollars "down the street."

3. *Your people will be more creative and innovative.* People who are having fun look at life and its challenges through different lenses. They see opportunities often missed by people who are just putting in time.

4. *Your patients will notice.* Being a patient in a professional office is stressful enough without being around a bunch of stressed-out staff members. Fun reduces stress for everyone. Patients enjoy coming to a fun-loving professional office, eagerly accept more treatment recommendations and refer their family and friends.

A prerequisite for having fun is a well-developed sense of humor. Some professional offices appear to have had a complete humor by-pass operation. However, the condition is not terminal. Following are six steps to a great sense of humor.

Six Steps to a Great Sense of Humor

1. *Have a core belief that the world is a funny place.* Look at the world through a pair of humor-enhancing glasses.

   From there to here, from here to there, funny things are everywhere.
   - Dr. Seuss

2. *Think funny.* Look at the flip side of all situations, especially when

Laughter is the most inexpensive and most effective wonder drug. Laughter is universal medicine.
- Bertrand Russell

When a thing is funny, search for a hidden truth.
- George Bernard Shaw

If I can get you to laugh with me, you like me better, which makes you more open to my ideas.
- John Cleese

things get tense. Ask yourself this question, "What could be funny about this situation?"

A practice without a sense of humor is like a wagon without springs — jolted by every pebble in the road. - Adapted from a quote by Henry Ward Beecher

3. **Add play to all the serious things you do.** Playful people do serious things better. Continually ask yourself this question, "How can we have fun with this activity and do a great job?"

Life is too important to be taken seriously. - Oscar Wilde

4. **Laugh with, not at.** We all have idiosyncrasies worthy of laughter. When you laugh with others about their idiosyncrasies, remember your own.

Humor keeps you in the present.
It is very difficult to laugh and be disassociated
with the people around you.
In that one moment together you have unity and a new chance.
- Alexis Driscoll

5. **Laugh at yourself.** Be a leader. Set a fun, contagious and healthy example for others.

Laugh at yourself first before anyone else can. - Elsa Maxwell

6. **Take your work seriously, but not yourself.** One of Southwest Airlines mottoes is, "Take yourself lightly and take your job and your responsibilities seriously."

The most revolutionary act one can commit in our world is to be happy.
- Patch Adams

A great way to add happiness to your office's day is to subscribe to our "Start Your Week with a Smile" program. We will e-mail, fax or mail you a page of humorous stories and jokes for you to distribute to each staff member every Monday. Call 800.917.0008 for a complimentary month of Start Your Week with a Smile.

Some Activities Other Dental Offices Do

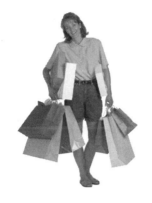

"One of our favorite ways to reward our outstanding team during the holidays is to take a Shopping Day. We work in the morning and take the afternoon off. We start by selecting a fun mall to take our team to, but we keep it a secret. The suspense is part of the enjoyment. We rent a limo or a motor home, stock it with snacks, soda, glasses, napkins, plates and a pizza. We eat on the way! When we arrive, we give each team member an envelope with cash. The amount varies with the length of service, but it's usually around $150.

We then review the three rules for the afternoon:

1. They must spend all of their money.

2. The money must be spent on themselves only.

3. They must be willing to show all of their purchases to the team.

After shopping, we gather back in the limo, have refreshments and participate in a 'show and tell.' Everyone 'oohs and aahs' and has a great time. The next stop is dinner at a favorite restaurant. This is a fun event that our team greatly looks forward to." – Drs. Gerald Bird and Dr. Jay Johnson, Cocoa, Florida.

"We decorate our bulletin board each month. Each employee takes one or more months during the year and decorates it according to the events of the month." – Dr. Wes Teal, Loris, South Carolina.

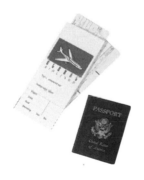

"We give special recognition for the team player who cheerfully gives 110 percent CONSISTENTLY. We give the employee two airline tickets to their favorite vacation spot." – Alan and Sandy Richardson, Spokane, Washington.

"One of the best ways to promote a better understanding of a parent's job is to provide a day for families to come to work and learn more about what goes on there." – Barbara Glanz, author, *Care Packages*.

"For the past six years, we've had a personal trainer come to our office three days each week. The exercise is great, and we have lots of laughs. It's fun, healthy and convenient. The office pays for one-half of the fee per session." – Dr. Harvey Kerstein, Clearwater, Florida.

"We do things together. We have an annual holiday party where all staff members are encouraged to bring their spouses and children. We also have an annual family trip to our local water park." – Dr. Bridgett Borris, Las Cruces, New Mexico.

"Our practice, in Woodenville, Washington, is known for its hot air balloon rides. We meet at 5:30 a.m. for a peaceful flight over our beautiful area. The touch down is a relief for some. The champagne toast awaiting us is a welcome treat for all!" – Dr. Michael Koczarski, Woodenville, Washington.

"Most everybody likes a 'new look.' Make appointments for your staff with an image consultant to help them with professional make-up and hair tips. This is an elegant approach if any of your staff overdo their hair and makeup." – Gary and NJ Miler, Columbia, South Carolina.

"We take our crew white water rafting after hitting our goals or after completing a difficult project." – Dr. Frank Adams, Greenwood, South Carolina.

"Our team loves to shop. Every year on the first weekend in December, we fly to San Francisco for three nights and two days of shopping. The office pays for the airfare, hotel and gives everyone $200." – Dr. Russell Kihara, San Diego, California.

Traveling with your team can be a big investment. More often than not, it's worth it because of the team spirit and memories created. Think about it. At the end of your life, are you going to remember the whole thing or just a few vivid experiences? Create memorable experiences for your team – and they will do the same for you.

Top Incentive Travel Destinations in the Western Hemisphere
(ranked in order of popularity)

1. Hawaii

2. Caribbean Islands

3. California

4. Florida

5. Mexico

6. Nevada

7. Arizona

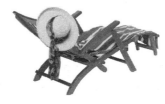

8. New York

9. Canada, Bermuda (tied)

10. Puerto Rico, Chicago (tied)

Top Incentive Travel Destinations in the World
(ranked in order of popularity)

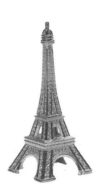

1. France

2. Spain, England, Germany, Italy (tied)

3. Australia

4. Portugal, Monaco, Austria, Switzerland, Hong Kong (tied)

5. Ireland, Singapore, Bali, Thailand, Israel (tied)

"We have a family night for the staff and their families at a professional baseball game – hot dogs, peanuts, popcorn and drinks for all." – Dr. Joseph Steiner, Charlotte, North Carolina.

"We schedule a 'ghost day' with fake appointments. When the staff comes to work, we take them water skiing, snow mobiling, bungy jumping or something else they would really enjoy!" – Dr. Bret Tobler, Provo, Utah.

"On Assistant's Appreciation Day in March, we take a limousine to a nearby city (in our case, Chicago) to have a fancy lunch and attend a show." – Dr. Marianne Kehoe, Geneva, Illinois.

"Once a year, coinciding with the Chicago Midwinter Dental meeting, our entire office stays at a hotel and goes to dinner and shows for three days and two evenings. This is a great morale booster for the entire office." – Dr. Martin Kolinski, St. Charles, Illinois.

"We had our staff show up in casual clothing for a planning session that was scheduled from 7:00 am to 6:00 p.m. When they arrived, we went to the airport for a flight to New Orleans. We shopped and roamed around Bourbon Street for the day." – Dr. Craig Smith, Atlanta, Georgia.

"Give the entire team a trip to a Glamour Shots to get both fun and staff photos taken. The office gives $99 toward each package purchased. Some of the photos can be used for a framed picture of the team for the reception room." – Drs. Stanley Allen and Drury Vincent, Greensboro, North Carolina.

"Hire a masseuse to give each staff member a 30-minute uninterrupted session just for them." – Dr. Tom Tomlo, Hendersonville, North Carolina.

"Give each staff member a make-over and color analysis." – Dr. James H. Maddox, Asheville, North Carolina.

"Give each staff member a coupon for an overnight stay at a local hotel with a jacuzzi and $50 to spend toward a romantic dinner." – Ed and Diann Crenshaw, Asheville, North Carolina.

"Surprise your staff by scheduling a fake 'day from hell.' Make the staff think that they are going to have to get through it all. Then at lunch, surprise them with the fact that the office has been very productive that morning; that you are on track for the month; and that they have the afternoon off!" – Dr. Tom Tomlo, Hendersonville, North Carolina.

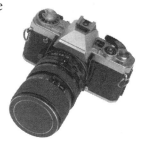

"Our office does a lot of socializing together. We always have a camera ready to capture the special moments. We put the pictures in a memories scrapbook and keep it in the reception room for our patients to see. It's a great conversation piece. We keep a second one with additional pictures that aren't appropriate to the patients." – Dr. Frank Adams, Greenwood, South Carolina.

"We picked five Fridays where we all worked without pay. Half the production went toward overhead and half of it went toward our Caribbean Cruise fund. Then all of us, including spouses, went on a cruise. It was awesome!" – Dr. Bud Evans, Chewelah, Washington.

Hold an office triathlon. Include the staff's families. Go to a family fun center, pick out three events that everyone can do (miniature golf, go-cart or bumper boat racing, skeeball, softball batting, etc.) and have a contests in various categories for the best "athlete." Give goofy prizes to the winners. Be sure to take pictures and put them in your office scrapbook.

Some More Activities You Can Do Together

Check the ones that appeal to you.

○ Have a caricature artist draw everyone's picture.

○ Show a comedy video (Mr. Bean, I Love Lucy, etc.) in the office over your lunch hour. Have popcorn, Milk Duds and red licorice vines for everyone.

○ Go to a midday movie.

○ Play miniature golf.

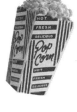

○ Go bowling.

○ Go to lunch or dinner on National Secretaries Day, etc.

○ Go sky diving.

○ Go scuba diving.

○ Take limousine ride "on the town" on Friday night. Pay for babysitting for your staff members with children.

○ Take a harbor cruise.

○ Take an ocean cruise.

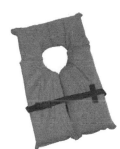

○ Go on a rafting trip.

○ Take a glider ride.

○ Take a biplane ride over the city.

○ Have a cookout or dinner at the dentist's home for staff, partners and kids.

○ Have a picnic or barbecue in the park for everyone. Pass out Frisbees with invitations attached to the inner side. At the picnic, pass out picnic kits with sun visors, sports bottles, bubbles for the kids etc. imprinted with your practice's name. This is a great way to thank people for extra time they put in on special projects.

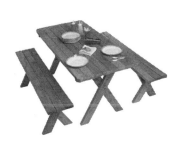

○ Have a Ferris Buehler Day Off. First, the entire office watches the video. Then, everyone takes the rest of the day off, hits the streets and does silly stuff they've always wanted to do – the more junior high-like the better. Everyone comes back at four o'clock and gives a report. The best story gets a convertible sports car rental for a weekend.

Take a second now to review this chapter. What ideas has it stimulated? What actions are you committed to taking in your practice? Write your answers in the space below:

○ _____

○ _____

○ _____

○ _____

○ _____

We covered a lot of material in this chapter, didn't we? Celebrations and activities are so powerful because they actively involve people. When people do things, especially with others, they vividly remember their experience. BE MEMORABLE! Make celebrations and activities a major part of your recognition and reward program.

Now it's time to move on to another important, and sometimes overlooked, component of an effective program. Read on to learn the power of . . . **Awards and Time Off**.

6 | Awards & Time Off

You learned about the fun-loving people at Southwest Airlines previously in this book. They're a superb example of a business team working together, in a complex service industry, to enjoyably achieve outstanding results. A interesting key to their success is found in their New York Stock Exchange ticker symbol. The symbol is LUV.

At Southwest Airlines, LUV is more than a symbol. It's a way of life. Here's what their Chief Executive Officer, Herb Kelleher, says about his people, "We are interested in people who externalize, who focus on other people, who are really motivated to help other people. We are not interested in navel gazers, regardless of how lint-free their navels are."

Southwest has two main engines that propel their love machine. First, they hire caring, loving people. Their motto is, "We hire for attitude and train for skill." Second, they treat their people with care, love and gratitude. They do this for three reasons:

To live without love is not really to live.
- Moliere

1. It's the right thing to do.

2. When you give care, love and gratitude, you will tend to receive love and gratitude.

3. Your staff will treat your patients the same way they're treated by you.

Sometimes dentists have a hard time using the words love and gratitude or showing these emotions in the office. They know it's important, but they think, "This isn't the place." Your staff's need for love and gratitude doesn't end when they walk in the office door. Many may be spending more time with their co-workers than they do with their own families. The essence of this book is not about giving stuff to people.

It's really about demonstrating love and gratitude to people – in many ways, at many times.

In this chapter, you will learn how to give these two vital emotions, love and gratitude, with awards and time off.

Awards

Awards should never be the primary component of your recognition and reward program. They can be effectively "sprinkled in." The following examples will show you how.

A Golden Attitude

"How do you develop a positive mental attitude in others? First, you need to set an example. If you're dejected and sullen, you cannot expect your co-workers to be excited and joyful. Attitudes are contagious. Make sure your attitude is worth catching. Second, recognize others who are setting a great example. A great way to do this is to give "golden attitude" pins to staff members who have a golden attitude toward your patients. Behaviors you will want to reinforce include: big smiles, rapport skills, focus on patient, cheerfulness, flexibility and a 'can do' spirit.

The pins are worn on their uniforms. They serve as a reminder that the team must have a golden attitude towards each patient and each other. When a staff member goes above and beyond her job duties, give her an additional golden attitude pin. When she gets a total of five pins, she receives a full-day spa treatment package." – Susan Simpson, Houston, Texas.

"We have a plaque in the reception area with the names of our staff members on gold name plates who have been with us five years or longer." – Dr. Martin Kolinski, St. Charles, Illinois.

Traveling Junk Trophy

Have a little fun with your awards by creating a "Traveling Junk Trophy." The trophy is really a piece of junk somebody "creates." The more obnoxious the better. The trophy is given to the staff member who gives an extra amount of care or love to a patient. When the recipient sees or hears about another staff member doing the same, she passes the trophy on at one of your team huddles or staff meetings. This is a great way to have fun and celebrate someone's good deed!

More Creative Ways to Use Awards

As you can see from the above examples, awards are more than just trophies and plaques. They are any symbolic item or gesture that tells people they're special. Here are some other ways you can give awards (Check the ones you're committed to using):

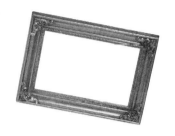

○ Place individual pictures of the staff on the reception area wall. Etch their names in bronze underneath.

○ Put one team picture on the wall in your reception area. Be sure people's names are underneath.

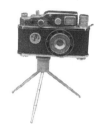

○ Place a book in the reception area with pictures of the staff, their families and a paragraph or two about the staff member's professional and personal life.

○ Put a team member of the year (or quarter) plaque on the reception area wall.

○ Buy and use preprinted certificates of appreciation purchased from an office supply store.

○ Buy a stuffed bunny and give it as the Energizer Bunny® Award.

○ Create a photo collage about a successful team project, showing the people who worked on it, its stages of development and its completion.

○ Mount patient "thank you" letters mentioning the staff members' names and hang them on your office walls.

○ Purchase trophies for staff members at a local trophy store. You will be surprised at the variety and uniqueness of the awards.

○ Request the Royal Scandinavia catalog. They have many elegant awards.

○ Create your own ABCD Award – Above and Beyond the Call of Duty. Present it whenever a staff member gives outstanding service.

○ Rent a billboard near your office. On it write, "To the greatest dental staff in the world!" Have all of their pictures and names included. Place your signature on the bottom.

○ Buy a full-page ad in your local newspaper with the same information as the example above. The employees of Southwest Airlines did this in *USA Today* in honor of their beloved CEO's birthday.

○ Use the Click and Print Motivational Software from Successories to create your own awards.

○ In many of the awards listed above, you can expand your team by including patients, vendors and families.

Add to the list
Answer this question, "What are some unusual or professional awards my staff would be honored to receive?"

○ _____

○ _____

○ _____

○ _____

○ _____

Time Off

Time off is another recognition and reward tool you can use. To many people, it's more powerful than money.

"It's fun to give when others are giving more than expected. As an example, when we have an intense project that takes us days to get done, we send people home early, buy them lunch and have fun – anything to lighten the load." – Alan and Sandy Richardson, Spokane, Washington.

"We give our staff time off with pay for meeting production goals. This motivates our staff to work more efficiently in less time. As a team, we determine a weekly production goal. Each week the goal is reached, the staff gets a future Friday afternoon off." – Drs. Debra Gray King and Richard Creasman, Atlanta, Georgia.

"As a group, we created a bonus system that involves time off with pay when a goal is achieved. Interestingly, this has been just as meaningful to the group as a financial bonus." – Dr. Paul Kuhlman, Corunna, Minnesota, FUNdamentals of Outstanding Teams.

"Occasionally, our staff earns an extra day off. We do this by giving them a calendar with the day X'ed out with a large, red mark and a big "Thank You" written on the date. Planning the day off near a weekend makes it even more appreciated." – Ed and Diann Crenshaw, Asheville, North Carolina.

Following are more creative ways to give your staff time off:

○ up to one year maternity leave with no or partial pay

○ a Friday or Monday off around a weekend holiday

○ an extra half-day or day off during the holidays for shopping or being with the family

○ a three-day weekend for no reason at all

○ a week off during the winter

○ flextime, if appropriate

○ a one-month sabbatical after ten years of service

○ 30 extra minutes at lunch

○ a week of two-hour lunches

○ a day off for their birthdays taken anytime within 30 days

○ an extra break during the day

○ a three-day weekend at the doctor's cabin or condo

Here are more creative ways to give your staff more time in their lives:

○ Hire someone to wash their car in your parking lot.

○ Hire someone to change their car's oil in your parking lot.

○ Hire someone to take care of their lawn for the summer.

○ Hire someone to clean their home for three months.

No person will have occasion to complain of the want of time, who never loses any.
- Thomas Jefferson

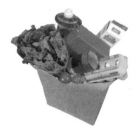

○ Hire a personal shopper to do their holiday season shopping.

○ Hire a concierge to run their errands for a month.

○ Hire someone to do their food shopping for a year.

○ Hire a babysitter to watch their kids for a weekend.

Does your brain feel like it's overloaded? If it does, that's OK. The key is to unload some of the information right now. First, briefly review this chapter. What ideas has it stimulated? What actions are you committed to taking? Now complete the unloading process by writing your answers below.

○ _____

○ _____

○ _____

○ _____

○ _____

Another extremely powerful way to create a sense of "we" in your office is to construct a compensation plan that rewards everyone for the office's success. Read on now to learn how to build . . . **Creative Incentive Plans**.

7 | Creative Incentive Plans

Almost every week you can pick up a newspaper or magazine and read about the millionaires being created through stock options given by corporations to their employees. Home Depot recently reported that over 1,200 employees became millionaires through their company share holdings. The stories of Microsoft, Starbucks and various internet companies' employees becoming wealthy are legendary. As you can see, it's not just the people at the very top of organizations that are cashing in. In professional practices, stock options usually aren't a reality; incentive bonuses, however, are an option.

The world is definitely changing. Dentistry is changing. The way people approach their work is changing. When it comes to compensation, people's expectations are changing. From the employees' point of view, the old rule of the compensation game was, "I'm thankful for my job. I work hard for and appreciate my salary. I expect raises based on my number of years of service." The new rule is, "If I do my best work, and my organization does well, I deserve part of the action. I expect compensation based on my degree of contribution and success of the business."

I'm not saying the new rule is right or wrong. I am saying it's a new game out there. It's important for you to know the new rules of the game so you can play the new game extremely well. If you play the new game with the old rules, you're going to be in for consistent disappointment. Personally, I like the new rules of the game. They inspire people to do their best work, which is a big difference from doing good work. The new rule may seem strange to you, but it's bringing back a healthy dose of self-reliance, which, in the long run, is good for everybody.

Of all the chapters in this book, this one is the least "buffet-like."

Economic incentives are becoming rights rather than rewards.
- Peter F. Drucker, author and management guru, from *1001 Ways to Reward Employees*

Creating an incentive plan can be confusing. I want to give you some clarity by featuring one proven plan – one that has been in place for years in thousands of professional practices. I want to thank Alan Richardson of Fortune Practice Management, Spokane, Washington, for providing the information below.

Five Steps to an Effective Incentive Plan

1. Base your incentives on net collections – not on production. Net collections are collections after refunds to patients and insurance companies.

2. Use a three-month running average to smooth out the highs and lows. Calculate and pay your bonuses on a monthly basis.

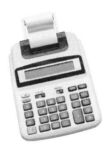

3. Determine what percentage of collections will be assigned to gross staff salaries. Gross staff salaries include any payments made to staff exclusive of other bonuses, pensions, well pay, vacation and holiday pay, medical and other benefit plans and pay to temporary staff. The percentage of collections assigned to staff salaries generally ranges from 20 - 25 percent.

4. Divide the number 100 by the percentage of collections assigned to gross staff salaries that you calculated in step three to create a factor. For example, 100 divided by 20 equals a factor of 5.

5. Using your three-month running average for net collections and staff salaries, complete the following steps:

   a. Total the prior three months' net collections. This number will be A in the equations below.

   b. Total the prior three months' salaries and multiply by the factor you created in step four above. This number will be B in the equations below.

   c. Subtract B from A. This will give you C. If C is a negative number, no bonus has been earned. If C is a positive number, a bonus has been earned. Proceed to the next step.

   d. Divide C by 3 to reduce to one month. This number is D in the equations below.

   e. Divide D by the factor you created in step four above. This number is your bonus pool.

f. Divide the bonus pool among your team members equally based on the number of hours they worked during the month. A part-timer who works half as much as full-timers receives half a share. The equations look like this:

A = Net collections

B = Three months salaries multiplied by your BAM factor.

A – B = C

C ÷ 3 = D

D ÷ factor = bonus pool

Bonus pool ÷ number of full-time employees = bonus pool share per full-time employee

For example, you have five employees who work 16 days per month and two who work eight days per month. The bonus pool is then divided by (5 x 16 + 2 x 8) = 96. If your bonus pool was $570.24, then each day's bonus would be ($570.24 ÷ 96) = $5.94. Those employees who worked 16 days would receive $95.04; those who worked eight days would receive $47.52.

Here is an example of how this works:

Assume that in April, May and June, net collections totaled $180,000 and total salaries for the three months were $30,000. We decided to use 20 percent of our collections for our salary costs, creating a factor of five.

Multiplying $30,000 by five equals $150,000, *subtracting* $150,000 from $180,000 gives us $30,000 to be divided by 3 (for the three months), i.e. $10,000. We then *divide* this $10,000 by the factor of five to get $2,000 (Bonus Pool).

Let's assume we have six employees – four who work four days per week, and two who work two days per week.

We total the days (or hours) worked in the previous month and *divide* the Bonus Pool ($2,000) by the total number of days or hours. For example, in the previous month the team worked 80 days total (64 days for the full-time staff, 16 days for the part-time staff). *We divide* $2,000 by 80, giving us a $25 bonus for each day worked. Each full-time employee earns 16 x $25 = $400, while each part-time employee earns 8 x 25 = $200. The four full-time employees receive a total of $1,600, and the two part-time employees recieve a total of $400, adding up to a grand total of $2,000 (Bonus Pool).

With this incentive plan, everyone wins:

1. Your staff wins because they see a direct link between their success and the success of the practice. Now, they will do their best work (and help their teammates do their best work) in order to achieve a bonus.

2. Your patients win because they will receive the best care from a team of excited professionals.

3. You win because you will receive a "bonus check" too. Part of the check will be emotional. Your enjoyment level will drastically increase because you will be working with a team of people who want to excel. Part of the check will be financial because there will be more money left over after the bonuses are paid.

Here are three things you can do to enhance the impact of the bonuses:

1. Pay the bonuses as close to the end of the month as possible.

2. Celebrate the distribution of the checks.

3. Each month, have a different staff member calculate the bonus and post the calculations in the staff room. This involves and motivates the team and removes all the mystery from the bonus plan. It's very important that your bonus plan is out in the open for your staff to see. If your staff links the bonuses to anything other than your practice's bottom line (favoritism, for example) all heck will break loose!

Following are two dentists' ideas on creative incentive plans:

"To reward my staff, I let them assume some ownership in the practice. I invite the staff to become aware of the business aspects of our practice. They must know that the era of entitlement is changing. Staff members are not entitled to automatic pay increases and promotions because circumstances keep changing. Instead of relying on their rights, the staff must take personal responsibility for their careers, embrace change and develop appropriate work habits for continued job success. The team must be ever mindful of ways to reduce costs and increase productivity. The amount paid for salaries and benefits (as related to total production and expenses) must be within the predetermined budget, which is established by me."

"If there's a surplus, I ask the staff how they want the excess money to be paid. I involve them in this decision. The options are numerous – a continuing education trip, a bonus or increased vacation time. Profit sharing transfers some of the risk of running a practice to the staff. They then have an opportunity to share in the rewards that accrue from their effort and favorable business conditions."

– Dr. David Jones, Cambridge, Ontario.

"My treatment plan presenter gets a monthly bonus based on three factors:

1. percentage of patients who accept the treatment plan and make a follow-up appointment
2. dollar amount of treatment patients have started in the previous thirty days
3. a subjective evaluation of the manner in which patients are being enrolled into the practice."

– Dr. Stephen Lawrence, Carlsbad, California.

I never worry about action, only inaction.
- Winston Churchill

Allow Your Practice to Bloom

Gardeners know that many types of flowers will go to seed and die if their blossoms aren't picked regularly. If the flowers are picked before they begin to fade and dry, more flowers will bloom and the plants will keep blooming throughout the summer, providing bouquets for friends and neighbors.

The same is true with the other joys and rewards of life. If we keep them to ourselves, they will dry up and die. If we share them with others, they will multiply.

Like all of the other ideas in this book, I hope you view a creative incentive plan as an investment, not an expense. An investment that will stimulate your team to be their best, do their best and give their best. Now your staff and you can have the best practice and all the rewards that go with it.

Ideas this chapter has stimulated:

1.

2.

3.

Now it's time to apply the information you've learned in this book to create a recognition and reward plan for your office. This is exactly what you will do in Chapter 9. If you're saying to yourself right now, "I'll just skip over this chapter and keep on reading." Or, "I'll get started with that next week." That means that you're the one who really needs to get started now! Often in life, the things you don't want to do are the things you need to do. Successful people do the things that unsuccessful people are unwilling to do. Be successful. Read and do the plan in Chapter 9 right now!

8 | The Power of Giving

From reading the previous seven chapters, I hope you see that a well-planned and effective reward program is really about giving. In this chapter, you will come to more fully appreciate the immense power that is released when a gift is given and received.

That power is increased as you move down the Four Levels of Giving described below.

It's not what we have, but what we give that brings joy.
- Anonymous

Four Levels of Giving

1. Level One - The receiver loses and the giver wins. The giver is a *con artist*.

2. Level Two - The receiver wins and the giver loses. The giver is a *martyr*.

3. Level Three - The receiver wins and the giver wins. The giver is a *true friend*.

4. Level Four - The receiver wins, the giver wins and other people win. The giver is a *team player*.

Level One: The receiver loses and the giver wins.
The giver is a con artist.

In reality, Level One isn't giving at all. It's taking under the guise of giving. All con artists take advantage of people by pretending to be givers.

Are there any areas of your life where you're unconsciously being a Level One giver? The feeling of guilt is a signal that this is happening.

Or other people may tell you that your "gift" doesn't feel like a gift. Remember, just because you think you're a giver, doesn't mean you are one. The receiver is the final authority of what is truly a gift.

The fantastic thing about an effective reward program is that your staff and you automatically win. You can't possibly be a con artist.

Level Two: The receiver wins and the giver loses.
The giver is a martyr.

Level Two is probably an improvement over Level One. The giver truly helps the other person, but gives so much or gives in such an inappropriate manner that he or she is hurt in the long run. This may seem admirable, but martyr-like giving decreases the ability to give in the future, because there is little left to give.

Sometimes parents who work outside the home fall into this category. They give to their spouses. They give to their children. They give to their employer. They give to their organizations. They give to their community. Then, at the end of the day, there is no time or energy left for themselves. They don't take care of themselves physically, emotionally or spiritually, which can lead to burnout or the "Is this all there is?" syndrome. The best thing these people can do is pull back on some of their giving so they have the ability to keep on giving in the long run.

You also may want to examine your life for any instances of Level Two giving. A sure sign of this is feeling unfulfilled after you give. I had this happen in my life about a year ago. As a speaker, trainer and consultant, I'm asked on numerous occasions to give complimentary presentations to not-for-profit groups such as Head Start, Job Corps, schools, prisons and civic groups. I was doing about twenty of these presentations a year. I love giving to these groups. However, on a long plane ride home from one of these presentations, I was feeling resentful about it. I'd been away from my family too much and I didn't feel good about that. I wasn't making much progress with this book and I was frustrated with that.

So I made the decision to limit myself to eight complimentary presentations each year. Three of them had to be in the San Diego area where I live. My decision has worked out well. I'm much more discriminating about who I do presentations for, and I feel good about each one I do. There will probably be a time in my life when I will want to increase the number, but for now, eight per year is the right number for me.

Another fantastic thing about an effective staff reward program is that when you give to them, you automatically win. You can't possibly be a martyr.

Level Three: The receiver wins, and the giver wins. The giver is a true friend.

In Level Three, there are no losers. The giver and receiver both benefit. With Level Three giving, both parties benefit because the act of giving provides energy to a series of events I call the Cycle of Life. The Cycle of Life is described in detail below. To make it more personal, let's make you the giver.

The Cycle of Life

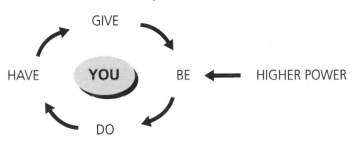

The Cycle of Life has four stages: BE, DO, HAVE and GIVE. Let's start with BE. When you use the words, "I am . . . You are . . . She is . . .", you are describing states of BE-ing. A person's BE-ing is like the juice inside a piece of fruit. Inside an orange is orange juice. When you squeeze (put pressure on) the orange, you automatically get orange juice. When you squeeze a lime, you get lime juice every time.

The same is true with people. When a person is an angry person, and the person is under pressure, you automatically get angry behavior. When you squeeze a loving person, you get loving behavior. When you are resourceful and happy, for example, you will do resourceful and happy things.

I also believe that there is a higher power who will give power to your BE-ing to energize your Cycle of Life. It's vital that you tap into this power source on a regular basis.

DO is the second stage of the Cycle of Life. You can DO mentally (think) or DO physically (take action). Much of your life is spent DOing things, but you have to ask yourself whether you're DOing the things that are meaningful, that will make a difference for others and yourself. If your thoughts and actions, your DOing, arise from empowering states of BE-ing, you will naturally choose to DO what is meaningful and important.

HAVE is the third stage of the Cycle of Life. Most people focus almost exclusively on the HAVE stage, and forget they need to BE and DO first! When you consistently DO the right things, you will HAVE the things you desire in life. You will HAVE all the relationships, emotions and possessions that accompany a life well-lived.

Now that you HAVE what you desire, you can't stop there – you must move to the fourth stage of the cycle. You must GIVE from what you HAVE. And more important than giving anything material, you must give to others your positive emotional states, like happiness and love. You must give away your support and knowledge. And yes, when appropriate, you may choose to give your physical assets as well. Your goal in giving should always be to enable the recipients to be more in their own lives. This is exactly what an effective recognition and reward program does.

Giving is a vital part of the Cycle of Life for two reasons. First, you will receive from life that which you give. When you give support, happiness and love, for example, you will receive support, happiness and love in your life because you will attract people and experiences that will enhance these positive emotions inside you. When you reflect a resourceful attitude to the world, you will attract the very resources you need – whether they are physical, emotional or spiritual – that will move you toward your personal vision. When you give happiness, you will attract it; when you give love, you become a magnet for all the love in the world. And these gifts of life will enhance your BE-ing, and the Cycle of Life can begin anew with even greater power!

You can also use the Cycle of Life when you want to BE, DO, HAVE or GIVE something in particular. As an example, if you want to BE enthusiastic, stop trying to BE enthusiastic. Instead, energize your Cycle of Life in each of the following four areas:

1. Tap into the energy of the Higher Power.

2. Mentally and physically DO enthusiastic things. Think about enthusiastic events in your life. Vividly focus on your dreams. Listen to motivational audiotapes. Put a big smile on your face, jump up and shout, "YES!"

3. HAVE enthusiastic friends around you. HAVE inspiring books by your bed. HAVE an occupation and/or hobbies that excite you.

4. GIVE your enthusiasm to others. Smile and talk to people you don't even know. GIVE enthusiastic compliments to people everyday. Enthusiastically GIVE support to other people who are moving toward their dreams.

When you do the above, your Cycle of Life will automatically create enthusiasm in your Being.

If you want to DO more high quality, comprehensive care in your dental practice, stop trying to DO that. Instead, energize your Cycle of Life in each of the following four areas:

I never worry about action, only inaction.
- Winston Churchill

1. Tap into the energy of the Higher Power. The Higher Power wants you to take action that makes the world a better place.

2. BE the kind of a person who would DO something like that. Model the people in your profession who are already DOing what you want to DO. What kind of DO-Juice they have inside of them?

3. HAVE the technical and people skills that will make it easy to accomplish what you want to DO.

4. When you're with your patients, come from a place of giving. GIVE them your knowledge, care and skill. GIVE them improved health and a more attractive smile. When you're with your staff, come from a place of giving. GIVE them the kinds of recognition and rewards that will improve their lives.

When you do the above, your Cycle of Life will automatically propel you to DO more high quality, comprehensive care in your practice.

If you want to HAVE a $200,000 income each year, stop trying to HAVE that income. Instead, energize your Cycle of Life in each of the following four areas:

1. Tap into the energy of the Higher Power. The Higher Power wants you to HAVE financial prosperity.

2. BE a professional who deserves a $200,000 income. Fill in the blanks in the following sentence, "I am a _____ , _____ , _____ and _____ dentist. As a result, I deserve a $200,000 income!" If you are having challenges doing the exercise, look at the people in

your profession who are earning that income and more. What kind of people are they?

3. DO mental and physical things that the $200,000 dentists DO. How do they think? Talk to them or listen to their audiotapes. Their conversations are full of clues. What are the core beliefs that drive their behavior? What activities do they DO every week? Success is not an accident. Success leaves clues. Model their behavior.

4. This may sound backwards, but to HAVE more money in your life, GIVE more money and time away. That's right, today, start giving more money and time than usual to your favorite charitable organizations. I'd also encourage you to DO something that I started doing a year ago. When you're in a restaurant or hotel, GIVE a person who rarely or never gets a tip a $20 bill. Smile, look them right in the eye, hand them the $20, and say, "I appreciate everything you do. Thank you." Then just walk away – no receipts for tax purposes, no preaching, just pure giving. You won't believe the opportunities that start coming into your life when you start doing this!

When you do the above, your Cycle of Life will automatically bring a $200,000 income into your life.

If you want to GIVE your family a nicer home, stop trying to GIVE them the home. Instead, energize your Cycle of Life in each of the following four areas:

1. Tap into the energy of the Higher Power. The Higher Power wants you to GIVE more.

2. BE the kind of person who would expect to live in a house like this. What empowering kinds of juice would BE inside this person?

3. DO the things a professional who lives in this house would DO. How many new patient exams would they DO each week? How much money would they collect each month? How would they communicate with their staffs and patients?

4. HAVE the income a person living in this house would have.

When you do the above, your Cycle of Life will automatically pay for the house of your dreams.

The bottom line is this, "When you want to BE, DO, HAVE or GIVE something in your life, focus on the other three areas in the Cycle of

Life and the Cycle will miraculously create that which you desire. The following says it best:

> *Happiness is like a butterfly.*
> *The more you chase it,*
> *The more it eludes you.*
> *But if you turn your attention to other things,*
> *It comes softly and sits on your shoulder.*
> - Anonymous

So, the first reason giving is a vital part of the Cycle of Life is that it jump-starts your Cycle. The second reason giving is a vital part of the Cycle of Life is that when you GIVE to others in empowering ways, they will never BE the same. You will help enhance their BE-ing, and a new improved Cycle of Life will begin for them, allowing them to DO and HAVE more-and GIVE more to others as well. Your Cycles of Life become interdependent. It looks like this:

The greatest good we can do for others is not to share our riches, but to reveal theirs.
- Anonymous

Interdependent Cycles of Life

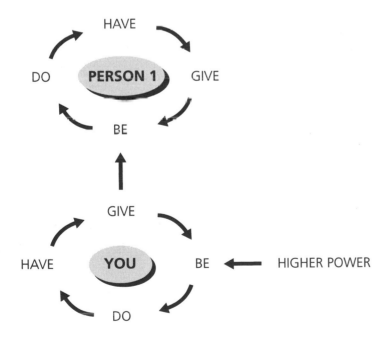

Level Four: The receiver wins, the giver wins and other people win. The giver is a team player.

Level Four is the highest level at which you can play the giving game. At Level Four, the receiver wins, you win and other people win. This is nothing more than connecting numerous Cycles of Life together to create one ever-expanding Upward Spiral of Life.

The Upward Spiral of Life

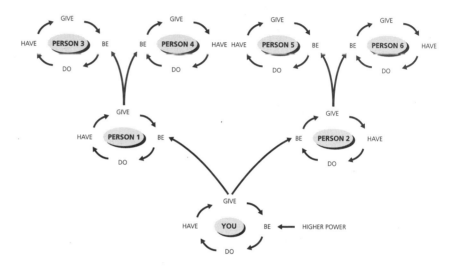

Here's a simple, yet revealing, example of creating an Upward Spiral of Life. As part of my travels, I take taxis in most cities I visit. I have two basic choices when I'm in the cab. I can ignore the driver and stay in my own world. Or I can have a meaningful conversation with the driver and learn from his or her experiences – which are almost always vastly different from my own. During the conversation I can always give the driver the gift of respect and appreciation. I ask about his or her experiences in life (often experiences gained in a different country). I ask for opinions of our country and us as a people. I ask, "What's one thing we Americans could learn from the people in your native country?"

At the end of the ride, I always give a nice tip, and just as important, I look the driver in the eye, shake hands, and say, "I appreciate the great service and the information you gave me." If they act interested in what I'm doing, I like to give drivers a copy of one of my books.

This is Level Four giving because:

1. The other person wins by receiving the gifts of respect and appreciation that enhance BE-ing.

2. I win. I enjoy seeing drivers come alive as they talk with me. You should see the change in their faces from the beginning to the end of the ride.

3. Do you think it stops here? How do drivers treat the next person in the cab? Perhaps a little bit better. How do they treat their families when they go home? Perhaps a little bit better. Maybe they'll even read the book to gain some knowledge that will make their lives and the lives of the people they care about better. In short, other people will win as a result of my gift.

When it comes to Level Four giving, you might be thinking, but there is so much I want to do. Where do I start? Start with yourself. As Mahatma Gandhi said, "Become the change you seek in the world." If you want to create a better practice, "Become the change you seek in your practice." Create a BE-ing who has enormous spiritual, emotional, physical and even financial riches. Tap into the Higher Power source everyday. DO the things that are needed. HAVE the skills, resources and emotions that are needed for success. Finally, create an attitude of giving. Look for places in all the professional and personal areas of your life where you can GIVE at Levels Three and Four on a consistent basis.

> Become the change you seek in your practice.

An effective recognition and reward program is a perfect example of Level Four Giving. When you reward a staff member, you win. Your Cycle of Life receives a jolt of energy. You will BE more enthusiastic. You will then DO better. You will HAVE more enthusiasm and financial resources. Now you can GIVE away that which you HAVE. The giving will enhance your BE-ing and your Cycle of Life will spin again with even more energy. You will literally BE on a roll!

When it comes right down to it, life is the flow of energy. When energy stops flowing in an organism or a dental practice, it dies. When more energy starts flowing in an organism or a dental practice, it becomes more vital. This principle applies to your life, your family, your organization, your community and your world. Giving is like a switch in your Cycle of Life. If you don't GIVE, the switch will turn off the energy and your Cycle of Life stops. When you do GIVE, the switch allows the energy to continuing flowing around your Cycle where it is amplified by your next act of giving. When you do GIVE, you pass the energy on to others, and they become "turned on." Now they can GIVE and pass on the energy to others, who can pass it on the others, who, well, you get the idea. Who knows how far it will go, how many lives will be touched?

I hope this book will be the spark that helps ignite your Cycle of Life, so your energy will flow with ease, creating a practice and a life that are ever-growing masterpieces of being, doing, having and giving!

9 | Creating Your Reward Program

Let's review what you've learned so far . . .

In *Chapter 1*, you learned the five reasons why rewards are vital to your practice:

1. In a time when fewer qualified people are available, staff-friendly professional practices are desirable places to work.

2. Younger people expect the workplace to be motivating and personally rewarding.

3. Coercion doesn't work over the long term. Sincere appreciation and rewards do.

4. A supporting and reinforcing environment fosters personal initiative.

5. Rewards are a low-cost way to encourage optimal performance.

You learned the nine guidelines for rewarding your staff:

1. Match the reward to the staff member.

2. Match the reward to the action or achievement.

3. Be specific. Let them know why the reward is being given.

4. Be timely. Give the reward quickly.

5. Use fixed and variable rewards.

6. Change your reward program frequently. Vary the who, what, when, where and why of your program.

7. Wrap every reward with emotion.

8. Create a formal reward program. Don't leave it to chance.

9. Begin with the end in mind. Crystallize your dream practice in your mind. Communicate your dream to your staff. Then put together a program that will help you get there.

In *Chapter 2*, you learned the five steps to an effective compliment:

1. Compliment the person as soon as possible after the behavior.

2. Begin the compliment with the person's name.

3. Compliment a specific action.

4. Explain why the action was important to you and the practice.

5. End the compliment by asking a question to gain more information or "tie a bow" on the conversation by saying, "Keep up the great work!" or, "I really appreciate having you on our team!"

You learned how to compliment your staff directly and indirectly through other people, how to be a storyteller and how to use your words, voice qualities and body language to add power to your communication.

You learned the three guidelines for using compliments to reinforce new behavior:

1. Don't wait for staff members to do it completely right before you compliment them. Compliment improvements.

2. Compliment people frequently at first. This is when they need the most reinforcement.

3. Decrease the frequency of the compliments as the action becomes natural.

You learned why recognition is so important and the five ways to multiply the recognition effect:

1. Include your office staff.

2. Include the staff member's family.

3. Include your patients.

4. Include your community.

5. Include your professional community.

Most importantly, you learned more than 50 ways to compliment and recognize your staff.

In *Chapter 3*, you learned that "full appreciation for work done" and "feeling included" were No. 2 and No. 3 on the list of ten things that employees value most from their jobs.

You learned that you can give gifts to:

1. acknowledge
2. praise
3. congratulate
4. celebrate
5. motivate
6. promote
7. thank
8. recognize
9. reward
10. cheer
11. apologize

You learned the seven keys to selecting the right reward item:

1. It is something the staff member desires.

2. It is useful.

3. It has a high, perceived value in relationship to its cost.

4. It has lasting value.

5. It is a highly recognized and valued brand.

6. It is appropriate for the reason given.

7. Its quality must reflect positively on your practice.

Most importantly, you learned over 300 ways to reward your staff with office logo merchandise, monogrammed merchandise, sports merchandise, electronics, general merchandise, food and clothing.

In *Chapter 4*, you learned that monetary rewards have weaknesses and strengths:

Finding unique gift items is easy!
Check out Appendix A for a complete list of resources.

Weaknesses of Monetary Awards
Monetary awards:

1. are not highly rated by employees as a motivator

2. don't motivate people to do their best work

3. have no lasting value

4. are not special

5. tend to become an expected reward

Strengths of Monetary Awards

Monetary awards:

1. can be given in doses during a long-term program

2. can be used as an incentive to inspire short-term behavior

3. can spark creative thinking

You learned the seven keys to using money as an incentive for achieving a short-term performance goal:

1. Set a realistic, achievable and measurable goal.

2. Clearly communicate what the monetary incentive will be.

3. Limit the time period to no more than three months.

4. Keep the rules simple.

5. Link the incentive directly to entire office or area of the office performance.

6. Involve as many people as possible.

7. Give the incentive promptly.

You learned how to use money to reward creative improvement ideas. You learned the four kinds of rewards:

1. Rituals - a holiday season bonus or a birthday gift

2. "Out of the Blue" rewards - any gift given just because you appreciate the person

3. Unanticipated rewards - flowers after a tough day

4. Incentives - a bonus for a goal achieved

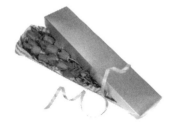

Most importantly, you learned over 75 ways to recognize and reward your staff with money and gift certificates.

In *Chapter 5*, you learned the four guidelines for preventing your staff from expecting rewards:

1. Use a variety of rewards.

2. Emphasize non-monetary rewards.

3. Link rewards to results.

4. Add emotion to each reward.

You learned the six benefits of celebration:

1. Celebration gives you a sense of history.

2. Celebration builds relationships.

3. Celebration helps you envision the future.

4. Celebration helps you recognize major milestones.

5. Celebration reduces stress and re-energize people.

6. Celebration creates enthusiasm.

You also learned the six guidelines for outstanding celebrations:

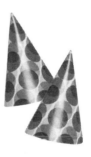

1. The celebration must be authentic.

2. The celebration must include as many people as possible.

3. The celebration must be fun.

4. The celebration must involve all the senses.

5. The celebration must be seen as an investment.

6. The celebration must be cost-effective.

You learned why it is so important to have fun at the office and the four benefits of fun:

1. Your office will be more productive.

2. Your office will have lower absenteeism and turnover.

3. Your people will be more creative and innovative.

4. Your patients will notice.

Most important, you learned over 110 ways to reward your staff with celebrations and activities.

In *Chapter 6*, you learned why love and gratitude are so important to your practice. Most importantly though, you learned over 40 ways to give awards and time off.

In *Chapter 7*, you learned why it's good business to provide economic incentives to your staff based on the results you achieve and how to construct a creative incentive plan that rewards everybody for the results your practice achieves.

In *Chapter 8*, you learned why giving is such an important part of your practice and your life.

In this book, I've presented over 555 Ways to Recognize and Reward Your Staff. (Have you been counting? It was actually 587.) Needless to say, you don't have to use all of them. You don't even have to think some of them are good ideas. The important thing is that you take action on some of the items you checked while reading this book.

This chapter will give you the blueprint to do just that in four easy steps.

Four Steps To Creating Your Reward Program

Step No. 1 - Begin With The End In Mind

As you learned in Chapter 1, it's not always advisable to start at the beginning. Many times it's best to begin at the end. Before you commence your reward program, crystallize in your mind the kind of practice you want to create. This is your dream practice. Your dream practice will be a beacon of light that will guide you in your reward journey. It will direct you to reward the appropriate steps on the path to your dream.

What is your dream for your practice? What would it look like? How would it feel? How many people will be on your team? How will the team members be treating each other? How will the team members be treating the patients? How many active patients will you have? What kinds of care will you be providing? What quality of care will you be providing? How will everyone feel at the end of the day? How many hours will you spend in the practice? How much vacation time will you be taking? What will be the financial rewards for the staff and you?

Take a minute or two right now to envision your dream practice. Shut this book and let your mind soar. Let the above questions stimu-

Action without study is fatal. Study without action is futile.
- Mary Beard

A rock pile ceases to be a rock pile the moment a single man contemplates it bearing within him the image of a cathedral.
- Antoine de Saint-Exupery

late your thinking. Don't be realistic. Realistic people accurately see the way things are now. Unrealistic people dream. They see things the way they could be and ask, "Why not?" All progress is made by unrealistic people.

Write a vivid description of your dream practice below:

Now that you have a description of your dream practice on paper, you need to do two things:

a. *Communicate the dream to your staff.* Vividly and passionately describe your creation. Ask for their help in creating it and construct a plan for them to share the rewards of the creation.

b. *Answer this question:* What actions and outcomes will move us toward that dream practice? These are the actions and outcomes you will want to recognize and reward. What are some intermediate goals your team will achieve on the way to your dream practice? These are the goals (financial and emotional) you will want to reward when reached. Here are some examples:

1. See 30 new patients a month.
2. Reduce our expenses by 7 percent.
3. Have a team that pulls together when things get hectic.
4. Increase our collections by 40 percent.
5. Have a group of people who all feel responsibility for the success of the practice.

The actions and outcomes that will move you closer to your dream practice:

1.

2.

3.

4.

5.

6.

7.

8.

9.

10.

11.

12.

13.

14.

15.

Step No. 2 - Set Your Budget

To start a successful reward program, four factors must be present:

1. *focus* - In a professional practice, there are many areas that demand your focused attention. Your reward program will not be successful

unless it is one of your top priorities. I hope the information in this book has made the establishment of a formal reward program in your practice a top priority.

2. *knowledge* - Not only do you have to have the desire to do something, you must have the knowledge to do it well. People who are just excited but don't know what they're doing are dangerous! I don't want you to be dangerous. Follow the guidelines presented in this book and you will have the knowledge you need to create a successful reward program.

3. *time* - It takes some time to create, administer and refine a reward program. This time can be invested by you or someone in your office who has the interest and skills.

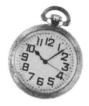

4. *money* - When setting a budget for your reward program, don't just think about how much it will cost. Think how much it will be worth to you! Many practices budget 2 - 3 percent of gross salaries for their programs. Remember that the most important part of your recognition and reward program costs nothing. You can also reduce the cost by bartering with vendors (preferably your patients). Another way to pay for bigger activities is to have the entire team donate their time. Remember in Chapter 5, the practice that paid for a Caribbean cruise for all staff members and spouses by working five extra Fridays.

My reward budget is $ _____ .

Step No. 3 - Create a Reward Plan

Review this entire book. Notice the items you checked and the notes you wrote. Use this information to create a reward program that moves you toward your dream practice and fits your budget.

On the following pages, record the ways you're going to acknowledge, praise, congratulate, celebrate, motivate, promote, cheer, thank, recognize and reward your office staff. You can use compliments and recognition (Chapter 2), merchandise, food and clothing (Chapter 3), money and gift certificates (Chapter 4), celebrations and activities (Chapter 5), awards and time off (Chapter 6) and creative incentive plans (Chapter 7).

The first page of your Reward Plan is for you to record the things you're committed to doing on a regular basis – things that aren't time sensitive. See a sample of this on page 105. Following this page are 12 monthly pages. In the first column on each page, write the date a particular reward will be given. In the second column, write the reward. In the third column, write the person or people to whom you're giving the reward. This could be the entire team. In the fourth column, write any notes that may be appropriate. This could be who is accountable for the item. How is the implementation of this item going to be monitored? See a sample month on page 106.

Things I'm Committed to Doing on a Regular Basis

Don't wait for next January to start. Begin with the month you're in right now!

1. If appropriate, compliment each member of the staff at least once a day.

2. Compliment my new chairside assistant, Maria, at least once a day when she makes an improvement.

3. Whenever I hear a compliment about a staff member from a patient, tell it to the staff member.

4. Add emotion to every compliment I give.

5. At least once every quarter, when any staff member goes "above and beyond," write a note to their spouse or parents.

6. At least once every month, leave a note, Post-it® Note, e-mail or voice mail thank you to every staff member.

7. Thank my people at every staff meeting.

8. If the last patient of the day doesn't come in, let staff know I appreciate them by letting everyone go home one hour early.

9. At the end of a tough day, give everyone a rose to take home along with my sincere thanks.

10. At least once a day, compliment a staff member by telling the patient the staff member did a wonderful job.

11. Use humor to break any tension that may build up.

12. Walk in the front door every day with a smile.

Things I'm Committed to Doing on a Regular Basis

1.

2.

3.

4.

5.

6.

7.

8.

9.

10.

11.

12.

Sample Month

Date	Recognition/Reward	Who	Notes
1	Energizer Bunny® Award	all	Pat buys it and start giving
1	recognition FUNdamentals	all	Pat order and start using when it comes
1	Bravo Board	all	Pat create and start using
4	birthday card to Belinda's son	Nick	Pat send
8	$5 per creative idea plan	all	I present at staff meeting
8	quarterly incentive plan	all	I present at staff meeting
16	go to lunch with Emily	Emily	I ask input to improve practice
17	go to lunch with Pat	Pat	I ask input to improve practice
18	go to lunch with Maria	Maria	I ask input to improve practice
19	go to lunch with Belinda	Belinda	I ask input to improve practice
23	dozen roses	Emily	Fifth anniversary with us – Pat buys
27	celebrate National Popcorn Day	all	Popcorn for all of patients and us – Pat buys
30	hot air balloon ride	all	Pat arranges

JANUARY

Date	Recognition/Reward	Who	Notes

FEBRUARY

Date	Recognition/Reward	Who	Notes

M A R C H

Date	Recognition/Reward	Who	Notes

A P R I L

Date	Recognition/Reward	Who	Notes

M A Y

Date	Recognition/Reward	Who	Notes

JUNE

Date	Recognition/Reward	Who	Notes

J U L Y

Date	Recognition/Reward	Who	Notes

AUGUST

Date	Recognition/Reward	Who	Notes

SEPTEMBER

Date	Recognition/Reward	Who	Notes

OCTOBER

Date	Recognition/Reward	Who	Notes

N O V E M B E R

Date	Recognition/Reward	Who	Notes

DECEMBER

Date	Recognition/Reward	Who	Notes

A good leader is one who approaches leadership as a calling,
a life engagement that, if done properly,
combines technical and administrative skills
with vision, compassion, honesty and trust
to create and environment in which people can grow personally,
can feel fulfilled, can contribute to a common good,
and can share in the psychic and financial rewards of a job well done.
- James A. Autry, *Love and Profit – The Art of Caring Leadership,*
from *1001 Ways to Reward Employees*

The above quote sums up this entire book. I hope you see why an effective reward program needs to be a vital part of the effective leadership Mr. Autry was talking about. I also trust you will take action today to create a recognition and reward program that will make your dream practice a reality.

In the next chapter, you will learn what to do after you've started your program. Find out how you can refine your reward program by reading through . . . **Frequently Asked Questions and Answers**.

10 | Frequently Asked Questions & Answers

Question: I know that rewards are important, but I'm having trouble making it part of my day. How can I do this?

Answer: This is the question I am asked the most. Here are five specific things you can do to make reward a natural part of your day.

1. *Do one thing differently for a week.* The next week do one additional thing differently. Don't try to do too much. You will get overwhelmed and do nothing.

2. *Make your staff part of your daily "to do" list.* That's where they belong anyway. Write the specific ways you are planning to praise and compliment each member of your staff.

3. *Get some help.* Maybe your office manager, spouse or interested staff member can take a major portion of the load off you. Be sure that everyone knows that you support the program 100 percent.

4. *Use methods of praise other than face-to-face.* It can be difficult to reward people in the middle of a hectic day. At the end of the day, sit back, relax and write a short note to your staff members and leave it at their work area. Keep a stack of note cards on your desk to remind you.

5. *Put four coins in your left pocket at the beginning of the workday.* Each time you praise a staff member, move one coin to your right pocket. This sounds corny, but it works. After you get in the habit, you won't have to do this anymore.

Free updates!
Get free updates to *555 Ways to Reward Your Dental Team.* Call 800.917.0008.

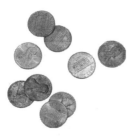

He who praises everybody praises nobody.
- Samuel Jackson

Question: Most of my staff is excellent. I have one person who is average. She does just enough to get by. Do I praise her?

Answer: The answer is, "Yes," if you want to keep getting average work from her and decrease the impact of your praise to your great staff members. Ken Blanchard says, "Nothing is more unfair than the equal treatment of unequals." The answer is a little more involved if you want to improve her work and maintain the great work of the other staff members. Keep praising the other staff members and let the average person know the specific improvements you would like her to make. Then praise any behavior that is a small step toward the improvement. Be sure to be sincere, specific and timely with your praise."

Question: I'm worried that any reward or incentive I give may become an entitlement. How do I keep this from happening?

Answer: Here are three great ways to keep this from happening.

1. *Link the reward or incentive to performance not presence.* A $250 bonus to everybody at the end of the year will be viewed as an entitlement after one year. Instead, set achievable goals and reward them when they are achieved.

2. *Vary your rewards and incentives.* This will keep the reward or incentive from becoming stale.

3. *Emphasize non-monetary rewards and incentives.* Revisit Chapter 2. It has over 50 ways you can recognize and reward with little or no money.

Question: I have one staff member whose performance seems to be getting worse as a result of the praise I'm giving her. She now has an attitude that she is better than everyone else. How can I correct this?

Answer: First of all, don't stop praising everyone else. When you see behavior you like, praise it. When you see behavior you don't like, give feedback. In this case, tell the person how their reaction to your praise is hurting their performance and relationship with the other staff members. When you see improved behavior from the person in these areas, praise that behavior.

Question: I don't seem to be getting any results from my program. What should I do?

Answer: The challenge is probably with your focus. What do you want to achieve exactly? What behaviors and results will move you closer to that achievement? Now reward these behaviors and results. Be specific. Don't reward everything. It's also possible that your rewards aren't desired by your staff. Check with them to discover what their motivators are. If at first you don't succeed, try something else.

Question: We have staff members of all ages in our practice. The younger ones seem to want different things from the workplace. Can you give me some insight here?

Answer: I think you will find the following generalizations extremely helpful. There are three age groups in the work force today. Each has different desires when it comes to working in a professional office.

1. *Mature workers were born between 1930 and 1945.* They are part of the "we" generation. As a result, these people tend to be very loyal and conforming. They are somewhat resistant to change and want predictability at work. Make sure they feel respected as a valued member of the team. Many of these people will work past retirement age if they can have flexible schedules or part-time hours.

2. *Baby Boomers were born between 1946 and 1964.* These people are part of the "me" generation. They grew up in times of economic prosperity so they expect a lot. They will work hard to achieve an incentive so they can buy more "stuff." Technology training is very important to them because they are feeling a little threatened by the younger workers who grew up with computers and high tech gadgets.

3. *Generation Xers were born between 1964 and 1981.* They are independent, resourceful and skeptical of authority. They want an exciting, challenging and fun work environment. They saw balance lacking in their parents lives, so their personal lives are more important than their careers. They want lots of skill development, tons of feedback, tangible rewards and fun, fun, fun!

Question: How do I measure the impact of my reward program?

Answer: There are three ways you can do this:

1. *Assess your staff's reaction.* Simply ask them how they think the program is going.

2. *Assess your staff's degree of behavior change.* Are they consistently doing the things that move you closer to your dream practice?

3. *Measure results.* What specific results did you want to achieve with your program? Are you moving closer to achieving them? Did you want to increase production or collections? Increase the number of new patients? Decrease overhead?

Question: What are some things we can do to keep our reward program fresh?"

Answer: Remember the nine guidelines for rewarding your staff in Chapter 1. If your program has gone stale, it's probably because you have gotten away from one or more of them. Here they are with my notes for actions you can take to refresh your program:

1. *Match the reward to the staff member.* Maybe what you're giving isn't what they want. Do a little detective work.

2. *Match the reward to the action or achievement.* Have a specific set of goals for your program.

3. *Be specific.* Let them know why the reward is being given. They must connect the reward to a specific action they took.

4. *Be timely.* Give the reward quickly. If too much time elapses between the action and the reward, the positive effect is diminished.

5. *Use fixed and variable rewards.* Don't become predictable.

6. *Change your reward program frequently.* Vary the who, what, when, where and why of your program. Variety is the spice of life!

7. *Wrap every reward with emotion.* No emotion leads to a cold and sterile program that drastically decreases effectiveness.

8. *Create a formal reward program.* Don't leave it to chance. Maybe you've let the administration and focus of your program slip a little.

9. *Begin with the end in mind.* Revisit your dream practice. This will show you the actions and results you want to reward.

About the Authors

Dr. Joe Blaes is America's most beloved dental editor. He is editor of *Dental Economics*, the nation's leading dental business journal, and *Dental Equipment & Materials*. He speaks regularly to dental groups throughout the United States and authors the widely read column, "Pearls for Your Practice." He can be reached at 314.434.6772 or *joeb@pennwell.com*.

Dr. Nate Booth is a communications coach, consultant and author of three best-selling books. Dr. Booth's mission is to "make dentistry fun." A frequent speaker to dental groups, he electrifies his audiences with his enthusiasm and humor. He is also the official spokesperson for Fortune Practice Management. He can be reached at 800.917.0008 or *nbooth@natebooth.com*.

appendix **A** | **Where to Locate Reward Items**

Argus Communications: Box 9550, Allen, TX 75013, 972.396.6500, *www.argus.com* PASS IT ON cards

Amazon.com: 1516 Second Ave, Seattle, WA 98101, *www.amazon.com* Books, videos, CDs and more.

Barnes & Noble: 100 Middlesex Center Blvd, Jamesburg, NJ 08831, *www.bn.com* World's largest bookseller.

Baudville Papers: 5380 52nd Street S.E., Grand Rapids, MI 49512, 800.728.0888, *www.baudville.com* Awards, certificates and cards.

Bennett Brothers Inc.: 30 East Adams Street, Chicago, IL 60603, 312.263.4800 Annual catalog with hundreds of gift ideas – many can be customized.

Best Impressions: 345 N. Louis Avenue, Oglesby, IL 61348, 800.635.2378, *www.bestimpressions.com* Unique promotional products.

Brielle Galleries: 707 Union Avenue, P.O. Box 475-V, Brielle, NJ 08730, 800.631.2156, *www.brielle.com* Twelve long-stemmed chocolate roses with silk leaves in florist box with red bow.

Borders Books & Music: 233 Winston Drive, San Francisco, CA 94132, *www.borders.com* Books, CDs and videos.

Brookstone: 17 Riverside Street, Nashua, NH 03062, 800.351.7222, *www.brookstone.com* Innovative gifts for home and office.

Bulova Corporation: One Bulova Avenue, Woodside, NY 11377, 800.423.3553 or 781.204.4600, *www.bulova.com* Solid brass miniature replicas of famous clocks. Customized watches that you can add one diamond per year by sending to Bulova. Sports team watches and clocks.

Carrot-Top Industries: 328 Elizabeth Brady Road, Hillsborough, NC 27278, 800.628.3524, *www.carrot-top.com* Flags and banners.

The Daily Planet: P.O. Box 64411, St Paul, MN 55164, 800.324.5950, *www.iloveadeal.com* Global clothing and gifts.

The Disney Store: 3805 Furman L. Fendley Hwy, Jonesville, SC 29353, *www.disneystore.com* Disney character clothing and gifts.

FLAX Art & Design: 1699 Market Street, San Francisco, CA 94103, 800.547.7778, *www.flaxart.com* Unusual art objects.

Franklin Covey: 247 Horton Plaza, San Diego, CA 92101, 800.416.1776, *www.franklincovey.com* Tools for highly effective living.

FTD: 3113 Woodcreek Drive, Downers Grove, IL 60515, 800.736.3333, *www.ftd.com* Flowers and seasonal floral gifts.

Hammacher Schlemmer: 9180 Le Saint Drive, Fairfield, OH 45014, 800.543.3366, *www.hammacher.com* Hard to find gifts and electronics.

Harry and David: P.O. Box 712, Medford, OR 97501, 800.248.5567, *www.harryanddavid.com* Gift baskets, fresh fruits, meats, baked goods and candies.

Historic Newspaper Archives: Hart Street, Rahway, NJ 07065, 800.221.3221, *www.historicnewspaper.com* Original date-of-birth newspapers back to 1880.

Idea Art: 2603 Elm Hill Pike, #P, Nashville, TN 37214, 800.433.2278, *www.ideaart.com* Promotional paper for desktop printers.

IntroKnocks: 16 W. 26th Street, New York, NY 10018, 800.753.0550, Extremely creative thank you cards.

Jackson & Perkins: 1 Rose Lane, Medford, OR 97501, 800.292.4769, *www.jacksonandperkins.com* Seeds, bulbs and flowers galore.

Lalique Crystal: 41 Madison Avenue, New York, NY 10010, 212.684.6338 Crystal vases, perfume bottles, etc. Can be personalized.

Lands' End Corporate Sales: 6 Lands' End Lane, Dodgeville, WI 53595, 800.338.2000, *www.landsend.com/corpsales* Office logo clothing.

Levenger: P.O. Box 1256 Del Ray Beach, FL 33447, 800.544.0880, *www.levenger.com* Tools for serious readers.

Longines-Wittnauer Watch Company: 145 Huguenot Street, New Rochelle, NY 10802, 800.451.2242, Watches and clocks. Can be personalized.

Movado: 610 5th Avenue, New York, NY 10019, 212.218.7555, *www.movado.com* Logo, personalized and add-a-diamond watches.

McArthur Towels: 700 More St., P.O. Box 448, Baraboo, WI 53913, 800.356.9168 or 608.356.8922, *www.mcarthur-towels.com* Monogrammed towels, robes and shirts.

Nightingale-Conant: 7300 Lehigh Avenue, Niles, OH 60714, 800.323.5552, *www.nightingale-conant.com* Motivational and inspirational audiotapes.

Northrup King Company: 7500 Olson Memorial, Golden Valley, MN 55427, 612.593.7333, Gourmet gardens in boxes.

Omaha Steaks International: Dept WB20, P.O. Box 3300, Omaha, NE 68103, 800.228.9872, *www.omahasteaks.com* Steaks and meat products.

Oneida Silversmith: One Seneca Street, Oneida, NY 13461, 315.361.3343, Personalized gifts, silverplate, stainless steel, lighting, gift boxed sets, entertaining items.

Open Please: Box 400 Centerbrook, CT 06409, 800.232.4244, *www.openpleasecatalog.com* Great ties, mugs, t-shirts, blankets, etc., all with dental themes.

Orrefors Kosta: 140 Bradford Drive, Bretlin, NJ 08009, 800.433.4167, *www.orrefors.se* Personalized, handcrafted crystal.

Nelson Marketing: 210 Commerce Street, Oshkosh, WI 54901, 800.982.9159, *www.nelsonmarketing.com* Imprinted promotional products.

Paper Direct: P.O. Box 2970 Colorado Springs, CO 80901, 800.272.7377, *www.paperdirect.com* Specialty papers, cards and presentation materials.

Parker Pen U.S.A., Ltd.: 1400 N. Parker Dr., Jamesville, WI 53545, 608.755.7000, Personalized gift pens.

Peet's Coffee & Teas: P.O. Box 12509 Berkley, CA 94712, 800.999.2132, *www.peets.com* Beautifully packaged coffees and teas.

Promotional Products Association: 3125 Skyway Circle North, Irving, TX 75038, PPA is an association of promotional products companies. Contact them for industry information or a list of distributors in your area.

Promotional Products Unlimited: 2291 W. 205th St., Suite 201, Torrance, CA 90201, 800.748.6150, *www.tromounltd.com* Huge selection of customized awards, pens, golf balls, watches, etc.

Royal Scandinavia: 140 Bradford Drive, West Berlin, NJ, 609.985.8740, Classic and contemporary porcelain, crystal, silver and stainless steel, executive desk items, unusual award items.

Santa's World Catalog, Kurt S. Adler Inc.: 1107 Broadway, New York, NY 10010, 800.243.XMAS, Over 20,000 Christmas items. Some can be personalized.

Seattle's Best Coffee: 1702-B Auburn Way North, Auburn, WA 98002, *www.seabest.com* Fresh roasted coffees.

Seiko: 1111 MacArthur Blvd., Mahway, NJ 07430, 800.545.2783, *www.seikousa.com* Personalized watches and clocks.

Sharper Image: 650 Davis Street, San Francisco, CA 94111, 800.344.4444, *www.sharperimage.com* Tons of great new gadgets.

Smith & Hawken: 1117 E. Strawberry Dr., Mill Valley, CA 949411, 415.383.4415, *www.smithandhawken.com* Garden tools.

Starbucks Coffee Company: 701 Fifth Ave., Seattle, WA 98104, 206.447.9934, *www.starbucks.com* Gourmet coffee and related items.

Starlight Originals: 11908 Ventura Blvd, Studio City, CA 91604, 800.726.9660 Unique bronze, pewter, and crystal sculptures.

Steel Threads: 1815 24th Street, Santa Monica, CA 90404, 310.998.1959, *www.stealthreads.com* Customized metal designs.

Success Builders: 600 Academy Drive, Northbrook, IL 60062, 800.231.2332, *www.baldwincooke.com* Hundreds of personalized items.

Successories: 2520 Diehl Road, Auroa, IL 60504, 800.621.1423, *www.successories.com* Click and Print Motivational Award Software, inspirational wall hangings, cards, plaques, and books.

Sugardale's: P.O. Box 571, Dept D, Massillon, OH 44648, 800.860.5444, *www.freshmark.com* Gourmet food items with personalized gift cards.

Sweet Nut Tree: 6210 Merger Dr. Holland, OH 43528, 800.477.6887, Gourmet nuts and candies in customized jars.

The "Red Plate": 4201 N.E. 34th Street, Kansas City, MO 64117, *www.waechtersbachusa.com* The "Red Plate" as described in Chapter 3.

Tiffany & Co.: 727 Fifth Ave., New York, NY 10022, 800.423.2394, *www.tiffany.com* Many low and high cost gift items that can be engraved. This is a great catalog!

Warner Brothers Store: Horton Plaza, San Diego, CA, 619.233.3058, *www.wb.com* Clothing and gifts with all your favorite Warner Brothers characters.

Waterford Wedgwood USA: P.O. Box 1454, Wall NJ 07719, 800.933.3370, China and crystal at various prices.

Wells Lamont: 6640 West Touhy Avenue, Niles, IL 60714, 800.323.2830, *www.wellslamont.com* Gloves with your logo.

Wilson Sporting Goods Co.: 8700 W. Brynmawr, Chicago, IL 60631, 800.432.0321, *www.wilsonsport.com* Golf balls, tennis balls, athletic shoes and bags personalized with person's or your office's name.

Wine Design: 4901 Morena Blvd, #307, San Diego, CA 92117, 800.201.9463, *www.vinodesign.com* Personalized wine and champagne bottles.

Wonton Food Inc., Fortune Cookie Division: 220-222 Moore Street, Brooklyn, NY 11206, 718.628.6868, *www.wontonfood.com* Fortune cookies with personalized messages.

Workman Publishing Co.: 708 Broadway, New York, NY 10003, 212.614.7509, *www.workmanweb.com* Unusual cookbooks, books, page-a-day calendars and traditional calendars.

Z Gallerie: 1855 W. 139th Street, Gardena, CA 90249, 310.527.6811, *www.zgallerie.com* Unique gifts and more.

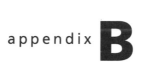

Dr. Nate Booth Learning Resources, Live Programs & Services

appendix **B**

Dr. Nate Booth Learning Resources

Do you want to learn more? Bring Dr. Nate Booth into your office via his highly effective video and audio programs and books.

Elegant Influence for Dentists

Does high quality, comprehensive dentistry sell itself? Not usually! You will increase your case acceptance when you can elegantly influence your patients to say "Yes!" to the treatment they deserve. The Elegant Influence Office Study Program contains eight audiocassette tapes, one video tape, five 93-page Learner's Guides (one for each staff member) and a Leader's Guide. In 10 action-packed staff meetings, your entire staff will listen to Nate Booth, DDS, and Brenda Kaesler, RDH, present the Seven Steps to Elegant Influence. The true power of the program comes next. Each staff meeting concludes with an Exercises for Action section where your team will practice the skills and develop a plan for using the skills in your unique office situation. The Elegant Influence Office Study Program is loaded with powerful communication skills you won't find anywhere else! Following are a few of the dynamic and effective communication strategies your team will learn:

- How to take fear out of influence so the patient and you feel comfortable with the process.

- How to naturally enter the patient's decision making process to help the person choose optimal dental health.

- How to create a reputation that sets the stage for easy acceptance of your treatment plans.

- How to discover the unique "buying motives" of each patient.

- How to use "Value Links" to connect the patient's "buying motives" with your treatment plan.

- How to elegantly ask patients to "open a relationship" instead of "close a sale."

- How to make the case presentation appointment an enjoyable and learning experience for everyone!

Eight Audiocassettes, Videotape, Leader's Guide & Five Workbooks - **$295**

The Diamond Touch: How to Get What You Want by Giving Others What They Uniquely Desire

We're all familiar with the Golden Rule, "Treat others in the way you would like to be treated." The Golden Rule is a powerful principle, but it has one shortcoming. Everyone wants to be treated differently. This variety of desires is what makes relationships interesting and challenging. The good news is the variety of desires creates tremendous opportunities for those people who understand and use The Diamond Rule. The Diamond Rule is, "Treat others in the unique way they want to be treated." Those who have The Diamond Touch quickly and precisely discover the unique desires of the people in their most important business and personal relationships. Then, whenever appropriate, these people give others what they want in the way they want it, to create close relationships that prosper and last.

In this enjoyable and insightful book you will acquire The Diamond Touch in the following relationships:

- Husband and Wife Relationships

- Service Relationships

- Parent and Child Relationships

- Friendships

- Work Relationships

- Influence Relationships

280 page hardcover book - **$25**

Jump Start Your Day

Each day you probably spend 15 - 40 minutes on your appearance so you can look good on the outside. How much time do you spend preparing emotionally so you can feel good on the inside? Most people answer, "Zero." Jump Start Your Day will help change that. In just eight minutes each morning, your entire team will learn to create the energy and enthusiasm you need to fly through your day with passion and purpose.

Two audiocassettes - **$25**

Thriving on Change
The Art of Using Change to Your Advantage

Rapid and never-ending change is a fact of life in today's world. What isn't a fact yet is how all this change is going to affect you! Some people live life at the mercy of change and avoid it at all costs. Others try to cope with change and just "hang in there." Change Masters are a different breed. They thrive on change! They know that rapid change levels the playing field and creates tremendous opportunities for anyone who knows the new rules of the game. In short, Change Masters use change to their advantage in their personal lives and businesses! In Dr. Nate Booth's refreshing and interactive book and audiotape, you will learn to create the future you desire and deserve.

333 page hardcover book - **$25**
75 minute audiotape - **$10**

To order, call 800.917.0008.
Or visit out web site at *www.natebooth.com.*

Dr. Nate Booth Live Programs

Bring Dr. Nate Booth to your group for a lively keynote presentation, a dynamic half-day seminar or an educational full-day training program.

Comfortable Influence
How to Enjoyably Influence Patients to Say, "Yes!"

You can be the most knowledgeable and caring professional in the world, with the best staff and outstanding services, but your impact will be severely limited if you a can't influence patients to take action on your recommendations. In Comfortable Influence, you will learn the psychological reasons behind why patients choose to take action. Now, you can naturally enter the process and comfortably influence them to say "yes" to your treatment plans.

You can schedule the Comfortable Influence Program in a keynote, half-day or full-day format.

Following are a few of the dynamic and effective strategies your group will learn:

- The three psychological principles that direct all behavior, and how you can use these principles in the influence process.

- How to create an identity that inspires you and influences others to take action.

- How to create a reputation that predisposes people to accept your recommendations.

- How to create an environment of trust and rapport.

- Three elegant ways to transfer emotion so that patients are excited about recommended treatment.

- How to elegantly ask the appropriate questions that comfortably lead to case acceptance.

- How to weld Value Links between your services and the patient's most compelling wants and needs.

- How to create urgency so that patients want to take the next step now.

- How to leverage yourself so that patients enthusiastically refer others to you.

Thriving on Change: The Art of Using Change to Your Advantage
Rapid and never-ending change is a fact in today's world. What isn't a fact yet is how all this change is going to affect your dental practice and you! Some people live at the mercy of change and avoid it at all costs. Others try to cope with change and just "hang in there." Change Masters are a different breed. They thrive on change! They know that rapid change creates tremendous opportunities for those who know the new rules of the game!

In changing times, the same set of beliefs, strategies and skills that have gotten your practice to where you are now will not get you to where you want to go. When things change, you must change. The thrill of running a practice or living a life is knowing what to change, what to keep and when and how to do each. In Thriving on Change, you will learn the skills needed to use any change to your advantage, creating greater success on all levels. You can schedule the Thriving on Change Program in a keynote, half-day or full-day format.

Following are a few of the dynamic and effective strategies your group will learn:

- The power of principles, and the habits they create, to shape your office culture and your life.

- The Six Thriving on Change Beliefs. These beliefs are the foundation of all successful change utilization.

- The success strategies dental practices and individuals use to harness the power of change.

- The Four Change Utilization Questions you need to ask to transform every change into an opportunity.

- The Three Keys to Anticipating Change.

- The Seven Steps to Creating Change.

- How to continually learn and grow so that you are smart, quick and flexible enough to consistently use change to your advantage.

The Diamond Touch: How to Give Patients What They Uniquely Desire

We're all familiar with The Golden Rule, "Treat people the way you like to be treated." The Golden Rule is a powerful principle, but it has one shortcoming – everyone wants to be treated differently! This variety of desires makes professional relationships interesting and challenging. It's also the reason why you can't take a cookie cutter approach to service in today's diverse and ever-changing world. The good news is this variety of desires creates tremendous opportunities for the dental teams who understand and practice The Diamond Rule. The Diamond Rule is "Treat others in the unique way they want to be treated." The dental teams who have The Diamond Touch quickly and precisely discover the unique desires of their patients. Then, whenever possible, these teams give the patients what they want, in the way they want it, which creates close relationships that prosper. You can schedule The Diamond Touch Program in a keynote, half-day, or full-day format.

Following are a few of the dynamic and effective strategies your team will learn:

- Why a "one-size-fits-all" relationship philosophy is doomed to fail in our highly individualized world.

- How to quickly "get on the same wavelength" with almost anyone you meet.

- The two questions you must ask to quickly and precisely discover patients' unique desires.

- How to use the Five Lifestyle Groups as a guide to applying The Diamond Touch.

- The four costly mistakes most people make when dealing with patients.

- Three 60-second strategies for dealing with difficult people.

- How to consistently get what you want in life by giving others what they uniquely desire.

The Power Of Synergy: One Plus One Equals Three

Remember a time when you were part of a synergistic group that was really "on a roll?" A group that worked together, magically became more than the sum of its parts, and created outstanding results? It was not an accident. There were Nine Keys to Synergy that led to your success.

1. The group must have a specific, well understood and common outcome.

2. The group must consistently stay in resourceful emotional states.

3. Team members must have specific and unique roles to play.

4. Team members must receive what they uniquely desire from an occupation.

5. The group must be constantly improving.

6. Team members must feel appreciated.

7. The group must communicate openly and well.

8. The group moves through challenges together.

9. The group must have outstanding leaders.

The Power of Synergy is designed to reinforce or create these essential elements of synergy in your professional team. With inspiring examples, proven synergy strategies and dynamic interaction, The Power of Synergy Program will help you build a dental team that is even more enjoyable, powerful, and effective! You can schedule the program in a keynote, half-day or full-day format.

Life Balance: How to Create a Life
That's Not Just Busy, But Well Lived

The demands on your time and attention are intense – work, family and personal time are all clamoring for your immediate attention. Congratulations: you're intensely wanted! The challenge lies in allocating the appropriate time and attention to each area of your life.

Life Balance will show you how to enjoyably get the right things done. Then, the end of the day, you'll feel the rewards of a life that's not just busy, but well lived! You can schedule the program in a keynote, half-day or full-day format.

In the Life Balance Program, you will learn how to:

- Crystallize what is truly important in your life.

- Consistently do the things that are important, not just urgent.

- Create balance and synergy among the various roles in your life.

- Jump off the "harder/faster/more" treadmill.

- Set and achieve balanced goals that produce quality results.

- Create a weekly guide that will assist you in enjoyably accomplishing the important goals in your life.

- Break the vicious cycle of procrastination and crisis.

- Make time for renewal of body, mind and spirit.

- Turn your days into an upward spiral of living and learning.

Creating Long-Term Results for Your Group

The above programs are not "one-time sessions" where your group feels good for a day and then its back to "business as usual." They are programs where your team will enjoyably learn practical, easy-to-use and effective strategies, and then want to take action to implement the strategies in their lives. Here's how:

- Each participant will receive a customized Learner's Guide, which they will complete during the program and then take home for reference and reinforcement.

- We will write an article for your association magazine or newsletter to be published after the program.

- If you desire, you can include as part of your program any one of our educational products that are designed to reinforce and enhance the information your group learns during the program.

For more information, call 800.917.0008.
Or visit *www.natebooth.com.*

appendix **C** | # Fortune Practice Management®

Have the Practice – and the Life – You Want

Imagine a scenario in which your office staff works like a well-oiled machine . . . Stress is at a minimum . . . your patient base is growing steadily . . . productivity and profits are up . . . you have time to spend with your family . . . to improve your golf game . , . travel . . . pursue a hobby . . .

An impossible dream? On the contrary. Whatever your vision, Fortune Practice Management can help make it a reality.

Take Charge of Your Practice

You honed your technical skills in dental school. But little did you know that in addition to DDS, you'd need to fill the role of CEO, CFO, Director of HR and VP of Marketing. Because today, being a dentist also means being a small business owner. In addition to providing top-notch patient care, you have to worry about profitability, personnel issues, training your staff, insurance, taxes, marketing and more. Chances are, all these extra responsibilities are eating into your personal time . . . time that would be better spent with your family or pursuing outside interests.

A Whole New Approach

Fortune Practice Management is a postgraduate training program that teaches dentists the essential business skills they need to run a profitable and thriving practice. Fortune provides an unparalleled combination of training, personal coaching, management and support systems designed to enrich the professional, personal and financial lives of dental practitioners. It is the only program of its kind in the country.

We Can Help You Build a Practice that Works

As a participant in Fortune's Management Program, you will learn how to develop a sound business plan, develop key management systems, lead and energize your staff and differentiate and market your practice.

The program begins with a comprehensive analysis of your practice, including a personal and financial goals and needs assessment. Once we've helped you define your vision for your practice, we work with you to develop a strategic plan for reaching your practice goals.

The Fortune Management Program will give you new control over your practice, enabling you to:

- Run your practice like a smart, successful business.

- Enjoy increased profits with less work and less stress.

- Experience measurable improvements in your practice.

- Create a more satisfying personal life.

Empower Your Team to Achieve Peak Results

The Fortune Practice Management approach encompasses every area vital to running a thriving dental practice, including:

- Internal and External Marketing

- Patient Relations and Exceptional Customer Service

- Appointment Scheduling

- New Patient Examination and Treatment Acceptance

- Patient Financial Management

- Preventive Maintenance and Recap

- Accounts Receivable and Collections

- Overhead Control and Profitability

- Personal Financial Planning

This team-based approach to training will result in a group of highly motivated professionals working toward the same practice goals. But don't think that the program is all work and no play. One of the secrets of our success is that we make the process fun – and memorable – for everyone involved!

Personal Coaching Focuses on Your Specific Goals

As a participant in Fortune's Management Program, you will be partnered with your own personal coach, who will guide you in applying the information and techniques you're learning. Between workshops you will participate in regularly scheduled phone calls with your coach. You also will receive a review and analysis of your practice's productivity and profitability indicators, as well as private, in-office consultations. The coaching sessions provide strategic advice tailored to your specific business objectives and provide guidance in these key leadership areas:

- Developing Your Essential Business Skills

- Managing Your Staff

- Overcoming Staff Resistance to Change

- Building a Motivated Team

- Holding Effective Staff Meetings

- Designing Staff Compensation and Bonus Programs

- Engaging Your Team in the Bottom Line

- Enhancing Case Presentation Skills

- Creating a Distinctive Level of Patient Service

- Hiring and Firing

. . . And much, much more

Take Better Care of Your Practice – and Your Patients

Professionals who have completed the Fortune Management Program tell us that their offices are happier places for their staff – and their patients. In a low-stress environment, you'll be able to focus on providing excellent patient care while increasing productivity and profitability.

Get Ready for a Life-Changing Experience

Professional Success. Personal Satisfaction. Financial Independence. You have the ability to achieve these things. Fortune Practice Management can show you how.

If you want to:

- Acquire the necessary business skills to develop a more profitable business

- Control your income level & the amount of time you work

- Be more productive

- Build a dental practice that works

- Have a more satisfying personal & professional life

. . . the Fortune Management Program is the best investment you can make in yourself, your business, your future.

Fortune Practice Management – Consulting with a Difference

Our commitment is to see you achieve the highest level of personal, professional and financial success. Our program combines the expertise of Anthony Robbins, the world's foremost peak performance coach, with the business expertise of Fortune's founding partners. It is this unique and balanced blend of business training and world-class motivation that sets Fortune Practice Management apart. After all, as one Doctor said, "It's one thing to provide business training for dental teams – it's another to get them excited to want to implement the information." That's what Fortune is all about. We invite you to experience the Fortune difference for yourself.

For more information, call 800.628.1052.
Or visit *www.fortunepractice.com.*

Bibliography

1001 Ways to Reward Employees, Bob Nelson, Workman Publishing, 1994. Absolutely fabulous book about rewarding employees. Much of the information is geared toward large corporations, but tons of usable information here.

Behavior Modification: What it is and How to Do It, Garry Martin & Joseph Pear, Prentice Hall, 1998. A comprehensive (464 pages), pricey ($60), and very valuable source of practical behavior modification information.

Built to Last – Successful Habits of Visionary Companies, James C. Collins & Jerry I. Porras, Harper Business, 1994. The best business book I've read in the 90s. Most of the concepts are directly applicable to your dental practice.

Care Packages for the Workplace: Dozens of Little Things You Can Do to Regenerate Spirit at Work, Barbara A. Glanz, McGraw-Hill, 1996. A fabulous book with numerous ideas you can use in your practice.

Changing Children's Behavior, John D. & Helen Krumboltz, Prentice Hall, 1972. The book is aimed at behavior modification for children, but same principles apply for adults. Believe it or not, it's still in print.

FUNdamentals of Outstanding Dental Teams, Vicki McManus, RDH, James & Brookfield Publishers, 1998. Excellent book on how to build a powerful dental team.

Funny Business – The Art of Using Humor Constructively, Bob Ross, Arrowhead Publishing, 1998. Useful book on humor in the workplace.

How to Run a Successful Service Award Program, Bulova Corporation, 1998, 800.423.3553. A concise booklet on the basics of service award programs.

How to Run a Profit-Building Corporate Gift Program, Bulova Corporation, 1998, 800.423.3553. A concise booklet on the basics of office gift programs.

Nuts! Southwest Airlines Crazy Recipe for Business and Personal Success, Kevin & Jackie Freiberg, Bard Press, 1996. A very readable book describing how Southwest Airlines enjoyably thrives in a very competitive industry.

The Best of Bits & Pieces, Economics Press, 1994. A useful book containing quotes and short stories on many topics.

The Diamond Touch: How to Get What You Want by Giving Others What They Uniquely Desire, Nate Booth, Harrison Acorn Press, 1998. This book will help you learn to discover what people truly desire. Now you can show them how to get it with your product, service or idea.

The 100 Best Companies to Work for in America, Robert Levering & Milton Maskowitz, Plume, 1994. Learn how the 100 best corporations in America treat their employees.

Thriving on Change: The Art of Using Change to Your Advantage, Nate Booth, Harrison Acorn Press, 1997. Learn how to harness the power of change to your advantage.

Walt Disney: An American Original, Bob Thomas, Hyperion Press, 1994. The best biography of Walt Disney.